Dr. G

Veterinary Laser Surgery
A Practical Guide

Veterinary Laser Surgery
A Practical Guide

Noel Berger
DVM, MS, DABLS

President, ex officio, Fellow
Veterinary Surgical Laser Society, LTD
Boston Road Animal Clinic, Inc.
Sutton, Massachusetts

Peter H. Eeg
BS, DVM

Executive Vice President
Veterinary Surgical Laser Society, LTD
Director of Small Animal Services and Laser Medicine
Poolesville Veterinary Clinic
Poolesville, Maryland

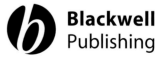

Blackwell Publishing Professional
2121 State Avenue, Ames, Iowa 50014, USA

Orders: 1-800-862-6657
Office: 1-515-292-0140
Fax: 1-515-292-3348
Web site: www.blackwellprofessional.com

Blackwell Publishing Ltd
9600 Garsington Road, Oxford OX4 2DQ, UK
Tel.: +44 (0)1865 776868

Blackwell Publishing Asia
550 Swanston Street, Carlton, Victoria 3053, Australia
Tel.: +61 (0)3 8359 1011

Authorization to photocopy items for internal or personal use, or the internal or personal use of specific clients, is granted by Blackwell Publishing, provided that the base fee of $.10 per copy is paid directly to the Copyright Clearance Center, 222 Rosewood Drive, Danvers, MA 01923. For those organizations that have been granted a photocopy license by CCC, a separate system of payments has been arranged. The fee codes for users of the Transactional Reporting Service are ISBN-13: 978-0-8138-0678-5; ISBN-10: 0-8138-0678-X/2006 $.10.

Original Graphic Art by Bob Feaster

Portions of Chapter 3 originally appeared in *Laser Surgery in Gynecology: A Clinical Guide*, (c)1993 Elsevier Inc. Reprinted with permission from Elsevier.

First edition, 2006

Library of Congress Cataloging-in-Publication Data available upon request.

The last digit is the print number: 9 8 7 6 5 4 3 2 1

To our families and colleagues
We strive to improve quality of life every day.

Contents

Foreword

Albert Einstein first described the concept of *laser* as an acronym for Light Amplification by Stimulated Emission of Radiation in 1917. It took more than forty years to pass before Theodore Maiman created the first laser, which was initially applied to surgical use. Since that time, lasers in medicine and surgery have widely expanded our abilities to more effectively fight disease and greatly improved our patient outcomes and comfort.

Laser techniques in oncologic surgery have become effective alternatives to radical tumor resection and to palliative tumor treatment methods.[1] CO_2 and Nd:YAG laser excision has been shown to provide almost a 50% improvement in the control of local disease in-vivo compared with scalpel resection in rodent mammary gland tumors and human oral mucosal lesions.[2,3] Lasers provide light with the necessary wavelength at the intensity sufficient for photodynamic therapy (PDT) for treating cancerous and non-cancerous lesions.[4,5] Specific laser wavelengths can be coupled to flexible fiber optics, which provides the possibility of improved surgical access via endoscopy, allowing for minimally invasive procedures and enhanced patient outcomes in the areas of upper respiratory, optic, gastrointestinal, genitourinary, and neurological surgery.

Despite the incredible development and advances that lasers have undergone in human surgical and therapeutic applications, lasers in veterinary practice have long been regarded as "surgical toys," given their expense and cumbersome size which made them impractical for private practice. In the past decade, however, technological breakthroughs have resulted in compact, portable, and reliable lasers that are economically feasible for both the general and specialty veterinary hospital. Laser use in clinical veterinary practice has become the newest "tool" for improved patient care and wider therapeutic options, but also poses additional health and safety hazards for the veterinary staff.

An understanding of laser light properties and interaction with tissue will result in optimal patient outcomes without increased risk to the surgeon, staff, or pet. For veterinarians to fully appreciate the advantages of laser energy, they must first understand how laser energy interacts with and affects living tissues before recommending or attempting to apply this technology to companion animals. The human literature has demonstrated these beneficial effects in lab animal studies and human clinical trials. These studies support the use of laser energy for the enhancement of quality of life and control of disease in the veterinary patient. They also provide a foundation for the commonly accepted laser surgical techniques and procedures which are constantly being implemented and refined in thousands of private veterinary practices around the world. Our pets can finally benefit from the very technology for which many research animals were used to perfect these laser surgical procedures on people. This book serves as a practical guide to the general and specialty veterinarian to understand and use laser energy in a safe and rational fashion to enhance our patients' quality of life and our overall standard of care.

Barbara R. Gores, DVM
Diplomate, American College of Veterinary Surgeons
Veterinary Specialty Center of Tucson
4909 N. La Canada Drive
Tucson, AZ 85704-1507
520-795-9955
brgdvm@aol.com

Notes

1. Paiva, M.B. et al. Nd:YAG Laser therapy for palliation of recurrent squamous cell carcinomas in the oral cavity. Lasers Surg Med 2002;31:64-69.

2. White, J.M., et al. Nd:YAG and CO_2 laser therapy of oral mucosal lesions. J Clin Laser Med Surg 1998;16:299-304.

3. Maker, V.K.; Elseth, K.M.; and Radosevich, J.A. Reduced in-vivo local recurrence with contact neodymium:yttrium-aluminum garnet (Nd:YAG) laser scalpels. Lasers Surg Med 1995;111:290-298.

4. McCaw, D. Photodynamic Therapy Can Successfully Treat Tumors. Vet Pract News 2001; 23.

5. Lucroy, M.D. Photodynamic therapy for companion animals with cancer. Vet Clin Small Anim 32 (2002) 693-702.

Preface

Laser light is a unique, extremely powerful, and very selective form of energy with the unparalleled ability to do beneficial work on living tissue. How it interacts with and changes living tissue is the central point to which many specialties strive to understand laser energy. For any veterinarian to have a full appreciation of the power that laser energy can have on their patients' quality of life, they must first understand the many physical and technical nuances that interrelate to provide this energy form. Laser energy can be applied directly to target tissue or administered to distant lesions at a remote site through fiber optic components. Each wavelength of laser energy has its own specific interaction with target tissues. Veterinary clinicians must fully appreciate the variation in tissue interaction by specific laser energy wavelengths before attempting to apply this technology to their patients.

Surgical and therapeutic use of lasers began in human medicine in the early 1960s. Unlike many technologies, the size, reliability, and portability of laser units has improved so rapidly that they are both economically and practically feasible for the general and specialty veterinarian.

The growth of laser use in veterinary medicine has progressed in the opposite fashion to standard-held dogma of university implementation and general acceptance first, followed by private practitioners' usage and acceptance. The ease of implementation and laser company tutorial courses have spawned a private general clinical usage and experimentation without great oversight from traditional educators. Only now are universities, at the request of laser companies and practicing veterinarians, securing and implementing lasers in their clinical protocols. It will still be some years before extended study and research into specific uses of laser energy already accepted by practicing veterinary clinicians will be verified in the traditional university study fashion. Anecdotally accepted techniques and procedures being refined and implemented in thousands of private veterinary practices in the United States and around the world will support the use of this type of energy system for enhancement of patient quality of life and relief of animal disease and suffering.

This book strives to help general and specialty veterinary practitioners both understand and implement the use of laser energy in a safe and rational fashion for the improvement of patient quality of life.

Acknowledgments

My first professional responsibility is always to focus on the welfare of my patients. When I first began experimenting with surgical lasers in 1996 I felt alone and in front of the pack with no one to guide me through the process. Fortunately, in a very short period of time, I was able to successfully perform surgical procedures for my patients more favorably. Immediately, my excitement grew and I felt driven to share my knowledge and experience with my colleagues. It was imperative that the veterinary profession should know what worked and what didn't. Seemingly invincible with lasers, I began using the tool for just about everything that I could do with a surgical blade or scissors. It was good, very good. My surgical cases were turning out better than ever before. I was able to approach surgical problems in an entirely different light! Now, I felt as though more complicated surgical cases were well within my abilities, and certainly after performing them successfully, my practice grew.

From an economic perspective, this has been one of the most exciting additions to my career. Laser surgery has allowed me to add more services that my practice can offer. My staff feels like they are special because they are part of a laser surgical facility, and they got to play with a lot of toys like video equipment and digital imagery as well as the laser and safety devices. Referrals from other veterinarians are common, and my career satisfaction has soared because I can help more patients, and I believe that I help them better.

This book is the result of many years of good experiences with lasers in surgery. My outpouring is the result of support from many friends and family. The desire I have is for every veterinary practitioner to be comfortable and competent in laser surgery. Hopefully this labor will help inspire you. There has been much effort by many to produce this work, and I wish to thank my lovely wife, Gayle, for giving me the freedom to learn and to teach. Also my three children Grace-Ann, Benton, and Samantha for never saying, "Daddy I miss you, please don't go," when I had to leave town to lecture or lead a wet lab. Also, my staff of laser technicians, especially James Koproski and Erik Bishop, for getting just the right shot when we needed to take a picture during a surgical procedure. Good Lord, thank you for giving me this life to share with others.

Noel Berger DVM, MS, DABLS

* * *

In preparing and compiling this book, I relied on my clinical experiences and independent research to gain an appropriate working laser program for my patients, clients, and clinical practice. I greatly appreciate the support of our technical staff, especially Candace Eck for her enthusiasm and common sense in supporting my clinical and surgical endeavors using laser energy. I must also give high praise to my wife, Cindy, and daughter, Jaime, for allowing their husband/father to spend great amounts of time traveling to lecture and learn about the potential of laser energy to improve patient quality of life. They also provided me with the luxury of private time at home in my office, putting my thoughts onto paper, to complete this book. I know they did it for all the animals in the world that they love as much as I do.

Finally, I hope my professional colleagues will use the information within these pages to refine and further expand the use of laser energy for the betterment of the veterinary profession and the improvement of their patients' quality of life.

Peter H. Eeg DVM

Part I
THEORY OF LASER SURGERY

Chapter 1
General Principles of Laser Energy and Biophysics

History

Light is one of the most interesting and mysterious elemental components of our known universe. It is intangible, yet able to transfer energy due to the mass effect of photons which enables light to do work and exert force on other molecules. Earliest man was in awe of light and held it as a gift from the gods. Great thinkers and scholars attempted to determine light's true origins and consistency. Modern science seeks to unleash its true hidden potentials for improving the quality of life on our planet.

Since the beginning of recorded time, light and the production of light has been used directly or indirectly to assist humans in their work. It has also been widely used in medicine, for instance to alleviate diseases such as rickets, reduce the painful effects of psoriasis, and more recently, aid in surgical intervention.

Photons, strictly speaking, are specific packets of electromagnetic energy that give light its mass and therefore allow it to do work. In 1905 Max Planck made this supposition in his equation $E=hf$, where E is the photonic energy, f is the electromagnetic wave frequency, and h is a constant (today known as Planck's constant). Equations were then developed that correctly identified the absorption and emission of black body radiation. Niels Bohr proposed a more closely related concept to that of today's laser energy in that this was related to a specific atomic model where electrons in specific atoms and molecules could alter their energy state to a higher or lower level, depending on energy applied, without being destroyed. In 1917 Albert Einstein recognized that a third emission form, stimulated emission, must also be in effect. This allowed theorists to reconcile differences between classical thermodynamic theorems and Planck's equation. While Niels Bohr's observations more closely reconcile true laser energy's potential, it was Einstein's consideration of the nature of stimulated photons, his unifying theories, that caused him to be credited as the father of modern lasers. These theories launched the quest for production of a coherent stimulated emission of radiation that would become known as laser energy.

This alludes to the idea that photons can be produced, amplified, and induced to cascade geometrically in a continuous positive feedback mechanism. It was technologically possible in the mid-twentieth century to prove the utility of selected materials for energy transformation. Simply applying electrical energy to a material caused the repeated release of photons, thus providing a new form of energy to do work. The first actual physical model for coherent stimulated radiation emission was in sophisticated microwave equipment developed to produce radar. Charles

Townes was credited as the creator of the MASER—microwave amplification by stimulated emission of radiation—and A.L. Schawlow provided the idea of an "optical type maser" or LASER—light amplification by stimulated emission of radiation—in 1958. It was Dr. Theodore Maiman, under the direction of Dr. Henry Gould, who successfully demonstrated consistent laser energy in 1960 with the production of a ruby crystal laser. Hence, a laser was realized in true physical form, placing both Bohr's and Einstein's theories into reality. The laser received its first use in veterinary medicine shortly thereafter, in 1964, in a laser-assisted vocal cord nodectomy.

Laser Physics

Radiation is the transmission of energy from one point to another with or without an intervening material medium. Electromagnetic radiation, which is produced by lasers, requires no medium for its transmission because it can travel through the vacuum of space. It can also travel through matter in the form of gases, liquids, or solids. The speed and direction of the propagation of radiation will be changed upon the transition from one medium to another in the form of heat.

Mechanical radiation is the transmission of vibrations through a material medium, e.g., sound. Sound travels quickest through dense media, and slower in more tenuous elements. The medium itself does not move as it conducts mechanical radiation; however, its particles oscillate about fixed positions, transmitting energy from one particle to the next in discrete waveforms.

A steady stream of particles such as electrons, protons, neutrons, etc., is also referred to as atomic radiation. No material is required for its transmission, but it can pass through various substances with some change in energy and direction. Atomic radiation usually requires a change in mass, and the energy transmitted is the kinetic energy or the moving particles.

There are two basic theories to explain the governing physics of electromagnetic radiation: the wave theory and the photon theory. Maxwell first described the wave theory in 1864. His theory describes the optical phenomena of visible light such as reflection, refraction, diffraction, interference, and polarization. It also describes the behavior of high-energy cosmic rays, X-rays, and other ultraviolet radiation as well as lower energy infrared, microwave, and radio waves. The wave theory does not adequately describe all of the behaviors of electromagnetic radiation, especially when dealing with high-energy reactions of nuclear particles. Planck modified the wave theory to describe the exciting discoveries of the photoelectric effect, light emitting diodes, fluorescence, photochemistry, and laser. His quantum theory, or photon theory, describes how materials can be stimulated to produce laser energy.

Light is generally described in terms of wavelength and frequency and travels at a speed, c:

$$c = 2.998 \times 10^8 \text{ m/s}$$

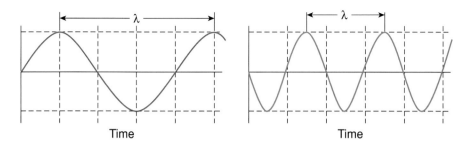

Time Time

Figure 1-1 At the same speed, c, frequency and wavelength are inversely related for these two different colors of light. The wave possessing a larger wavelength will have a lower frequency and less energy while the higher frequency wave will have a shorter wavelength and higher energy.

Wavelength is the physical distance between successive crests of waves of photonic radiation (Figure 1-1). The wavelength of light determines its physical characteristics. Visible light is perceived within a narrow band of wavelengths between 400nm (violet) to 700nm (red). Wavelengths shorter than 400nm are ultraviolet, and wavelengths greater than 700nm are infrared. Cosmic rays have the shortest wavelengths, on the order of 10^{-13} to 10^{-15} m, and radio waves have the longest wavelengths, up to one meter (Figure 1-2). The frequency of light refers to the number of wave crests passing a point during a defined length of time. The relationship between wavelength (λ), speed (c), and frequency (f) of light is given by:

$$\lambda = c / f$$

The wave theory of electromagnetic radiation describes each ray of light as composed of a combination of traveling waves of electric (E-wave) and magnetic (H-wave) fields. Each field is mutually perpendicular to the other and to the direction of propagation at all times. Each ray is composed of E-waves radiating outward in all possible planes, and for each E-wave there would be a corresponding H-wave perpendicular to it. The result is a ray of light composed of a waveform that resembles a string of pearls; the junction of the waves at the axis of propagation delimits the shape of each "pearl."

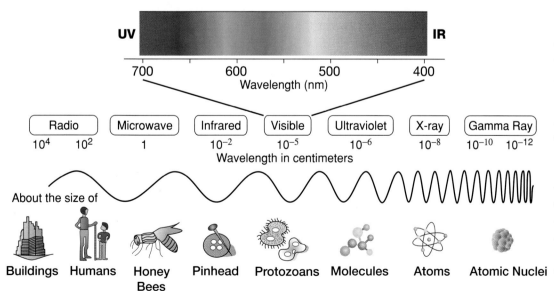

Figure 1-2 A simplified demonstration of the entire electromagnetic spectrum shows that visible light occupies an extremely narrow bandwidth. Red light is visible at around 700nm, and blue light is visible at around 400nm. Wavelengths larger than 700nm are referred to as infrared because the frequency of the radiant energy is lower than that of red light. Likewise, wavelengths shorter than 400nm are referred to as ultraviolet because the frequency of the radiant energy is higher than that of violet light.

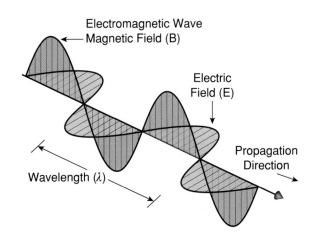

Figure 1-3 This is a simplified theoretical three-dimensional model of a photon of light. It indicates both an electric field and a magnetic field oscillating mutually perpendicular to each other and to the direction of propagation at all times.

Planck advanced the photon theory by postulating that the energy carried by an electromagnetic wave cannot be endlessly subdivided into ever-smaller increments, but that radiant energy consists of indivisible units referred to as a *quantum*. We now refer to this packet of energy as a *photon*. A photon is a massless particle of radiant energy that moves at the speed of light in a straight line. It may be considered a wave train of finite length, or a *wavelet*. Each wavelet is composed of a finite number of E-waves and corresponding H-waves bounded by a damped amplitude envelope (Figure 1-3).

The quantum theory states that there is a precise value of energy associated with each photon. The photonic energy (e_p) is directly proportional to the frequency (*f*) of the wavelet:

$$e_p = hf$$

$$h = 6.626 \times 10^{-34} \text{ Js} \quad \text{(Planck's constant)}$$

Since $f = c / \lambda$, photonic energy increases inversely with wavelength, and proportionally to frequency. Thus, ultraviolet radiation is inherently more energetic than infrared radiation. Although a photon has no mass, it does have the equivalent of momentum and can exert force on an object and transfer its energy. Einstein first suggested that photonic energy could be harnessed to perform work. He postulated that the basic substance of matter and energy are interchangeable, and are related by:

$$e = mc^2$$

The quantum theory of atomic structure also allows only certain electron orbital sizes, shapes, and distances from the atomic nucleus (Figure 1-4). It predicts that negatively charged electrons are found within *shells*, as a cloud surrounding the positively charged nucleus. These permitted orbits may be spherical, elliptical, conical, or a combination of these geometrical shapes. Furthermore, there are discrete levels of energy that an electron must possess to inhabit any particular orbit. Each atomic element is characterized by a unique number of protons, neutrons, and electrons. If the protons and electrons are unequal in number, the element is said to

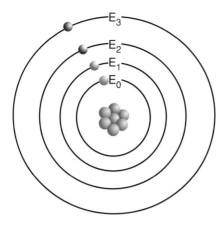

Figure 1-4 The nucleus of an element is a cluster of particles having a net positive charge. Negatively charged electrons inhabit orbital shells of definite size, shape, and distance from the nucleus. Higher energy electrons may inhabit higher energy shells at a greater radius from the nucleus. Orbits located closer to the nucleus may contain lower energy electrons. In this representation, E_3 is the highest energy orbital, and E_0 is the lowest.

be *ionized*. *Isotopes* of a given element have the same number of protons and electrons, but have a different number of neutrons; hence they have identical chemical properties. The *atomic state* of an atom is described by four quantum numbers:

- The principal quantum number, characterizing the shell of the electron (1 to 7), based on the radius of distance from the atomic nucleus
- The orbital quantum number, characterizing the orbital angular momentum of the electron (*s, p, d, f*); hence the shape of the electron cloud (Figure 1-5)
- The orientation quantum number, describing the direction of the electron cloud vector relative to an electric field (x, y, z, z2, x2-y2, xz, yz, xy); the orientation of *f* clouds is too complex to be described and is not salient.
- The spin quantum number, characterizing the angular momentum vector of electron spin as parallel or opposite to the orientation of the electron cloud (up or down). Therefore, either zero, one or two electrons may inhabit any given orbital at a given moment in time.

Electrons that orbit close to the nucleus have lower energies than those orbiting within higher energy level shells farther away from the nucleus. The value of the electron's energy is called its *atomic energy level*. The

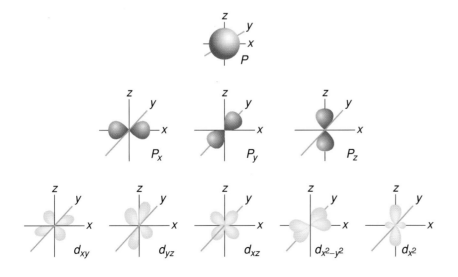

Figure 1-5 The number of possible orientations of atomic orbitals in space depends on the shape and size of the orbital. An *s* orbital is spherically symmetrical. There are three sets of bilobed *p* orbitals, and the axes along which the three orbitals lie are mutually perpendicular to each other. The five *d* orbitals are two sets of bilobed regions arranged in space as shown. Finally, there are seven *f* orbitals. Their shape and directional characteristics are not understood well enough to be shown.

quantum theory requires that the energy level change only by discrete increments of energy represented by the difference in energy levels of one orbit compared to another. Any change in the energy level of an electron within its orbit will cause it to instantly move to another orbit. This change occurs in distinct steps, and a continuous transition is not possible.

The quantum theory fundamentally describes how differences in photonic energy are related to changes in the atomic energy level. All light in the universe originates as a quantum-level energy change resulting in the spontaneous emission of a photon. Photons are generated and absorbed by molecules or compounds and have predictable energy levels. Each molecule has unique physical characteristics regarding absorption and emission of photonic energy. This emitted light is a characteristic wave of photons that can be collimated, amplified, or refined to transfer its energy to do work on a host of materials and tissues. Furthermore, the atom, molecule, or compound is not destroyed or used up in this process of photon generation. A variety of compounds, when stimulated, are able to produce differing wavelengths of laser energy. Each specific wavelength has a different effect on specific target material or tissue.

Laser light is distinctly different from other light in many ways. To illustrate, let us compare it with the "white light" produced from an incandescent light bulb (Figure 1-6). The product of the laser is light, which is composed of the previously described discrete energy packets known as photons. Photonic energy is also released from heat generated through resistance to a metal coil in a light bulb and indeed, a photon is a photon whether it comes from a camp fire, a light bulb, or laser. Light from the laser and the light bulb differs fundamentally in how its photons are generated, organized, confined, and transmitted. When you look at a glowing light bulb, you see white light that is composed of various wavelengths radiating in all directions at varying amplitudes and frequencies at all origins of time. As you walk away from the glowing glass bulb, its light appears dimmer until the light is no longer detectable. The various wavelengths produced from the light bulb cancel each other out over time and

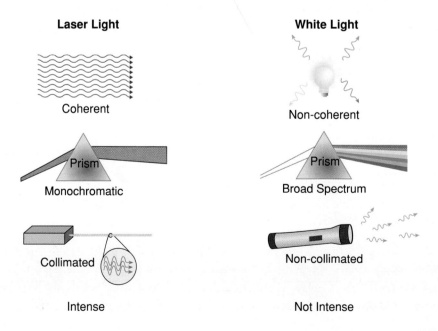

Figure 1-6 Laser light is coherent, monochromatic, collimated, and intense. Note the differences between laser light and the white light produced by an incandescent light bulb.

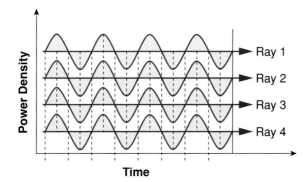

Figure 1-7 Coherence is demonstrated using these four photons. All of them have the same wavelength and velocity. There is coincidence in the peaks and troughs of the radiant energy, and they all begin at the exact same moment in time. Note that as the number of photons increase, the intensity, or power density, of the laser beam increases.

distance. In the laser beam, however, photons are emitted in parallel and in phase with each other and collimated. Photons produced from a single compound or atom producing consistent energy released at the same wavelength, amplitude, frequency, and time are considered a laser beam. This property is known as coherence (Figure 1-7). It allows the photons to maintain a stable wave pattern that permits the light formed to maintain collimation over great distances, conserving its energy potential. It also is able to maintain its ability to do work or impart its energy to a target material or tissue over an infinite distance. The intensity of a collimated laser beam is not diminished over distance.

We can also see that a light bulb produces a "white" color. This is because the white light contains all of the colors and wavelengths in the visual portion of the electromagnetic spectrum. Multiple photon emission of this nature is considered polychromatic. If you put a glass prism in front of the light bulb, you will refract the different wavelengths and see the rainbow effect spread out as a continuum of distinct color emissions. Laser energy passed through the same glass prism will produce light of only one wavelength and hence one color. A laser produces a beam of one type of photon and is classified as monochromatic.

A third difference between the two light sources is their intensity. The number of photons produced by a laser in a measured specific unit area is a much greater source of energy than for any other light source. This concentrated energy delivered to a compact area gives lasers the potential to do a huge amount of work.

Finally, it is important to note that although all photons obey the same basic laws of physics within the universe, the preservation of matter makes a laser quite distinct from a consumable light bulb. The concept of a cascading, reusable, and consistent supply of photons that are coherent, monochromatic, and intense requires an atom, molecule, or compound that can repeatedly alter its electrons in the ground state to a highly excited state and back without losing any of its own mass.

Laser Generation

Three things are needed to produce a functional laser: (1) an *optical resonant cavity* that contains (2) the lasing *medium* and (3) an *external energy source*. The type of lasing medium (gas, liquid, or solid) within the optical resonator determines the wavelength of laser light produced. The

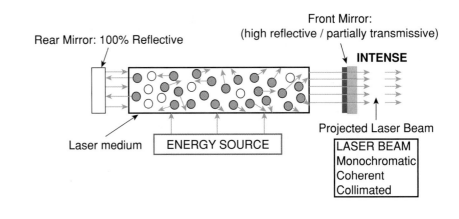

Figure 1-8 The capability to generate laser light is produced only by certain media contained within a resonant cavity following strong pumping by an external energy source. Stimulated atoms emit photons in all directions at first, but when population inversion occurs, axially oriented photons amplify geometrically to produce an intense, monochromatic, coherent, collimated beam of light. This photon cascade event occurs within pico-seconds, and is sustainable as long as energy is applied to the system. Some laser media are obligated to be pulsed by energy to exist. Laser energy is released from the resonant cavity through a highly reflective/partially trans-missive gate. The user may now harness laser light to perform work.

resonant optical cavity is generally a tube or cylindrical structure, and its length is much greater than its width. A highly reflective mirror caps one end of the resonant cavity and a partially transmitting but highly reflective mirror is at the opposite end cap. This is required to allow the laser light to emerge from the resonator for functional use. The energy source can be another laser or, more commonly, electricity (either radio frequency or direct current). The process of exciting the medium within the resonator is called *pumping* (Figure 1-8).

In a laser system, atoms in the ground state are excited by the input of energy to the resonance chamber. The electrons jump to a higher energy level called the singlet state, which is very unstable. Very shortly afterward a small amount of non-photonic energy is released, allowing the electron to move down to a meta-stable state. An atom in the meta-stable state can be stimulated by a photon to release two more photons, creating a geometric cascade effect of photon generation. According to the basic principles of quantum physics, since both photons come from identical energy levels, they will be the same wavelength (color) and move parallel to and in phase with each other. The release of this additional energy allows the molecule to return to a lower energy state. At a lower level, the atom can be repeatedly excited and stimulated to emit photons. When the process ceases, the electron returns down to the ground state by a non-radiative transition.

Only certain types of atoms or molecules are capable of what is referred to as repeated photon emission or the "lasing process" that will be described in greater detail in the following paragraphs. These atoms, molecules, or compounds can be in the form of a solid, gas, liquid, crystal, or plasma. Media suitable for laser generation are unique in that these atoms can remain meta-stable for a relatively long time, upwards of a couple of seconds or more. That is a lifetime in the physical world of the atom, compound, or molecule, where most reactions occur in nanoseconds or picoseconds (Figure 1-9).

Absorption and Emission

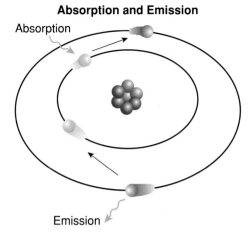

Absorption

Emission

Figure 1-9 Most reactions at the atomic level occur within a fraction of a picosecond. The absorption of energy by an atom causes an electron to jump to a higher energy level. This change in energy can be calculated using modifications of Planck's law, $\Delta e = hf$. Likewise, when an electron moves to a lower energy level it spontaneously emits energy in the form of a photon equivalent to that change in energy level.

The laser medium must be held in a sealed container. Within a fraction of a second, there is an intense buildup of many photons in a limited space. The generated photons are parallel and in phase with one another. This rapid production of intense, coherent photons is called a *photon cascade event*. It is repeatable and sustainable as long as the same energy input exists. Within the closed container, opposing highly reflective surfaces allow the photons to continuously reverberate through the excited medium. This allows for stimulating the emission of more photons, as was discussed earlier. This is the final physical process known as *photon amplification*. By causing the photons to continually re-enter the molecule mix, they enhance the production of more photons of the same wavelength. Then, controlled laser emission is produced by guiding the release of some of the photons by means of one partially reflective surface at one end of the laser cavity and passing them through an aperture. The result is the production of an intense, monochromatic, coherent, collimated beam of laser light.

Quantum Theory

An atom will normally exist in the ground state, corresponding to its lowest possible level of energy (Figure 1-10). It can rise to a higher level only in discrete steps, by absorbing energy in quantum increments. After absorbing energy, an atom exists in an excited state (Figure 1-11). The atom will return to a lower level excited state after a short period of time, and finally return to its ground state by emission of energy. This emission can take the form of a series of wavelets, or a photon, and the process is referred to as spontaneous emission. The frequency of the photon is:

$$f = c / \lambda = \Delta e / h$$

where Δe represents the change in energy between the excited level of the atom and the lower level to which it returns by spontaneous emission (Figure 1-12). The value of this energy change is usually expressed in joules or electron volts and they are related as follows:

One eV = 1.6022×10^{-19} J

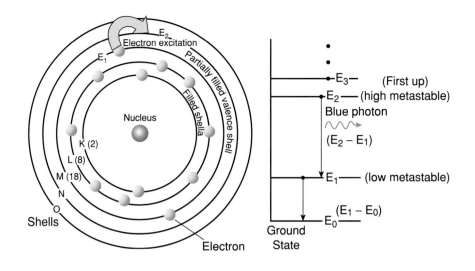

Figure 1-10 A representation of the possible atomic energy levels that can exist within a single element of a laser medium. The ground state, or E_0, exists at rest. When this atom is excited, an electron will jump up to the First Up level, or E_3, then almost immediately move to a slightly lower energy level E_2 (high metastable state). This energy state is not stable, and if no further excitation occurs, the electron will move down to a lower energy level (low metastable state), E_1, and radiate a photon by emission of energy equivalent to that change in energy (E_2—E_1). If no further excitation exists, after a very short period of time the electron will return to the ground state. Energy changes associated with E_3—E_2 and E_1—E_0 are usually lost as heat. The fundamental characteristic of any laser medium is the physical property of possessing a meta-stable state (E_2—E_1) that can be maintained for measurable periods of time.

Stimulated emission is the basic process that produces the phenomenon of all lasers (Figure 1-13). It occurs when an excited atom is irradiated by a photon that was spontaneously emitted by another atom of the same element, relaxing from an identical excited state. This photon causes the excited atom to emit an identical photon and return to a lower energy level. The original spontaneously emitted photon and the new photon emitted by stimulated emission are identical. They have the same wavelength and frequency, and are coherent in time and space. Amplification of light at

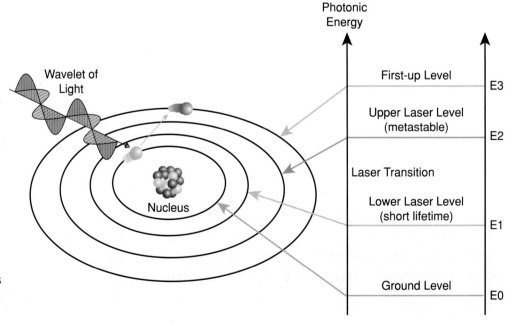

Figure 1-11 The absorption of energy, *e.g.*, a wavelet of light or photon, causes an electron of this atom to move up to a higher energy level state.

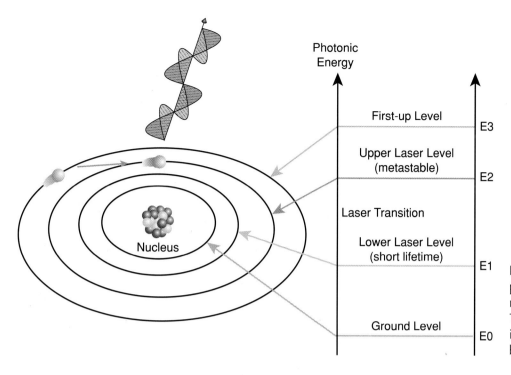

Figure 1-12 Spontaneous emission of a photon occurs when an excited electron moves down to a lower energy orbital. The wavelength of light emitted is inversely related to the change in energy between these two levels.

this frequency occurs as a geometric chain reaction within a resonant cavity. As a result, laser occurs.

At the atomic or molecular level most media have at least three, but more commonly four, distinct quantum levels of energy that are considered in the discussion of laser generation. The lowest level is the *ground state*, in which the electrons are closest to the nuclei and have a low energy level. When the medium is pumped, an electron absorbs sufficient energy to inhabit the *first high level*, or singlet state. Very shortly thereafter,

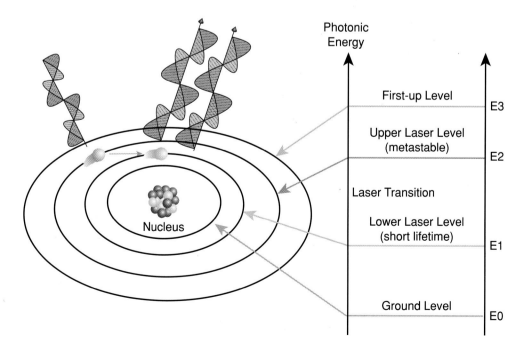

Figure 1-13 An excited atom can be stimulated to emit radiation as illustrated. An incoming photon triggers a second identical and coherent photon to be emitted parallel and in phase to it while simultaneously causing an electron to move from the upper metastable laser level to the lower metastable laser level. The photonic energy of the triggering wavelet is equal to the energy change ($\Delta E = E2 — E1$). The atom in the low meta-stable laser level may be excited again or it may return to the ground state by a non-radiative transition if no further energy input occurs.

the electron spontaneously falls to the *upper laser level* and the element or molecule is considered in a *meta-stable state*. The wavelength of the emitted radiation is determined by the change in energy between the upper and lower energy levels of the meta-stable state. This change in energy is known as the *laser transition*. Following emission of radiation, the electron falls to the ground state. The pumping cycle can begin again after the electron falls back to the ground state by a non-radiative transition (Figure 1-14).

When the concentration of a medium within the resonant cavity is high enough, it is more likely to create an environment conducive to laser generation. The photons released as a result of stimulated emission will be generated in an infinite number of directions. These randomly oriented photons will be absorbed by other atoms within it, creating stimulated emission of photons. Only those photons that are oriented perfectly parallel to the axis of the resonant cavity will continue to be reflected back and forth without a change in direction. If this axially oriented photon interacts with an electron in the ground state it will be absorbed and the laser effect diminished. In great contrast though, the true chain reaction of laser light generation is intensified if this photon aligned with the axis of the resonant cavity interacts with an excited electron residing in the meta-stable state. The result is that many photons will all simultaneously reflect over and again between the end caps of the resonant cavity in perfect alignment of space and time, creating a cascade of photons containing the same wavelength, frequency, and direction of motion.

For a continuous laser effect to occur, it is essential that the external energy source for pumping provides a condition in which the majority of individual electrons are in an excited state. It is also vital to maintain the meta-stable state for a reasonable period of time. Since excited electrons very rapidly return to a lower level, it is desirable to choose a medium that has a meta-stable state lifetime significantly longer than its ground state. Only certain media have these physical properties. The accumulation of molecules or elements that exist in the meta-stable state is necessary to sustain conditions contributing to laser generation. This requirement is referred to as a *population inversion* or *photon cascade*. Only when a population inversion exists can a laser sustain its action. The end result of laser is an intense beam of single wavelength (*monochromatic*) light that

Figure 1-14 Only media that can be sustained in the meta-stable state for appreciable periods of time are suitable for use in laser light generation. While pumping is maintained by electric current, triggering photons causes a geometrically increasing population of coherent light waves. In these conditions, an electron may repeatedly oscillate between the upper and lower laser levels, releasing a stimulated photon in each cycle. Amplification of coherent, monochromatic, collimated light within a resonant cavity by the stimulated emission of radiation is laser.

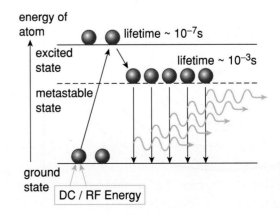

is in phase with respect to time (*frequency*) and space (*coherent*) and is confined within a determined boundary (*collimated*).

Beam Geometry

Collimated beams of light are parallel to one another in all three dimensions. The photon paths neither converge nor diverge at any time. When a laser emits light, the beam is collimated. This beam of laser light is also coherent, meaning all the crests and troughs of the waveform line up. Spatial and temporal coherence of all photons of laser light implies that at any point in the future, the position and intensity of that photon can be predicted; likewise, it is possible to determine the exact previous location and intensity of a laser photon by knowing its present position. The third fundamental characteristic of laser light is monochromaticity, or being composed of one constant wavelength.

Laser light output is described in terms of energy (joules), power (watts) and their respective densities. Energy is the measure of excitement of a substance that allows work to be performed and is expressed in joules. Power is the ability to do that work over a given period of time and is expressed in watts. Laser energy dosage delivered to an area is described in terms of fluence, or energy density, and is expressed in joules/cm². The very important concept of "power density" refers to the amount of energy delivered to a given area per unit of time and is expressed in watts/cm².

Energy is expressed in Joules

Power = Energy / Time

Fluence = Energy / Area energy is applied

Power Density = Power / Area power is applied

The cross section of a laser beam is generally circular, but the power density varies somewhat across its diameter, depending on the transmission device (Figure 1-15). This is largely due to the slightly curved shape of the reflecting mirrors within the resonant cavity that concentrates photons into the center of the beam. It is generally therefore most powerful at the center of the beam, and that power exponentially diminishes toward zero away from the central axis. Thus, a plot of power density vs. distance from the beam axis would be a Gaussian distribution pattern, which is described by:

$$P_r = P_a \, e^{-2(r^2/w^2)}$$

where P_r is the power density of the beam at radius r away from the central axis of that beam, P_a is the power density at the exact center of the beam, e is the base of natural logarithms, and w is the radius equal to one-half of the *effective diameter* of the beam. The effective diameter of a laser beam is the diameter of a concentric circle perpendicular to the axis of

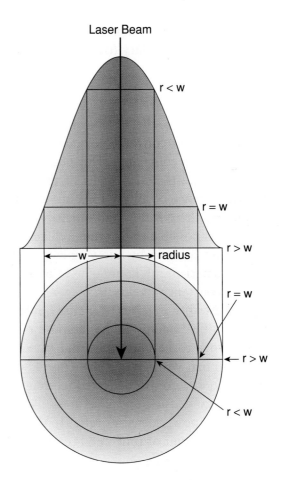

Laser Beam

r < w

r = w

r > w

w radius

r = w

r > w

r < w

Figure 1-15 The geometry of a TEM$_{00}$ laser beam is Gaussian and 3-dimensional. The highest power density, P$_c$, is at the center of the beam. Power diminishes logarithmically (Gaussian curve) with distance from the central axis. The effective diameter of the laser beam is represented by a cross section at radius r = w which defines an area equal to 86.5% of the total spot. Here the power P$_r$ = P$_a$/e^2. It follows then, that at radius r < w, the fluence will be much higher than at the edge of the laser beam, and at radius r > w the fluence will be very low.

travel of that beam, containing 86.5% of its total power. A simple calculation shows P$_r$ = 0.135 P$_a$ when *r* equals *w*. Thus, 13.5% of the beam's power lies beyond this radius that defines a circle containing 86.5% of the power of the beam.

The distribution of power density across a laser beam is called the *transverse electromagnetic mode* of the beam, or TEM. Many distributions of power density are physically possible and are designated as TEM$_{mn}$ where *m* and *n* are positive integers representing the number of troughs in the x-direction and y-direction of a three-dimensional plot of the intensity profile of a beam traveling in the z-direction (axis). Thus, a Gaussian beam has TEM$_{00}$, and a beam designated by TEM$_{01}$ would appear to be a bell-shaped dome having a deep central crater at the apex, appearing much like a typical volcano. Complicated TEMs are rarely desirable in surgery, and the most common useful mode of any laser beam is TEM$_{00}$, or the *fundamental mode*.

Laser photon output can be altered via a variety of mechanical and computer-assisted formats with modern lasers. If a laser delivers radiation continuously, it is operating in *continuous wave mode* (CW) (Figure 1-16).

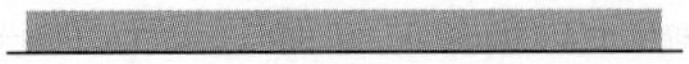

Figure 1-16 In continuous wave (CW) mode, the laser output is steady and constant for the entire duration of the time that it is used. Duration of CW operation may be as short as a few milliseconds, or indefinitely, and causes the greatest accumulation of heat within tissues.

Figure 1-17 In pulsed-wave mode (PW), the laser output is cyclically interrupted according to mechanical settings chosen by the user. The frequency of pulse repetition, f, can be as few as 1 Hz or as much as 50 Hz or greater. The time period of the radiant output, T_p, is the same during each pulse, and the rest period when the power is shut off, T_r, is also the same during each pulse. Some laser media are obligated to function in pulsed mode since the meta-stable state is not indefinitely maintainable. All lasers that function in CW mode can be used in PW mode. Using a laser in PW mode allows for some tissue cooling between pulses.

There are also user-defined settings for a laser to be operated in a series of timed pulses or *pulsed-wave mode* (PW) (Figure 1-17). This is also sometimes called a *chop wave mode*. Some lasers are restricted to pulsed-wave operation due to the physical properties of the medium, which prevent continuous laser operation; *e.g.*, excimer, Er:YAG, Ho:YAG, and ruby are all lasers restricted to PW operation. Lasers such as alexandrite (or any other diode), argon, CO_2, and Nd:YAG are capable of CW output, but can be operated in a pulsed mode. Superpulse and ultrapulse are specific waveforms that can be used in CO_2 laser systems either continuously or in a pulsed pattern (Figure 1-18), and will be discussed in Chapter 4. Several means of achieving a pulsed operation are known and used via a variety of programmed settings. They include *pump-pulsing, mode-locking, Q-switching,* and *cavity dumping,* just to name a few.

Pump-pulsing is achieved by intermittently interrupting the flow of power from the pumping source into the laser resonator by a mechanical, electric, or shutter switching device that is usually pre-programmed. This is the most common way a CW laser operates in PW mode. Mode-locking, Q-switching, and cavity dumping are all methods that create a large burst of laser energy extremely rapidly within the resonant cavity. The power is not long lasting, though, and the process is cyclically repeatable. Lasers that operate only in PW usually require pumping in one of these three ways to function. Mode-locking generally produces laser output in pulses on the order of 10^{-9} to 10^{-12} second. Although the energy per pulse may only be as small as a few millijoules, the power delivered

Figure 1-18 The superpulse mode (SP) of laser delivery is created using extremely short T_p and a corresponding longer T_r per pulse. The peak power is also much higher than a pulse of energy delivered by CW. The total fluence delivered by SP is generally lower than that of CW or PW. Ideal delivery and rest allow for the longest possible thermal conduction within tissues while maximizing tissue penetration due to high power densities achieved during T_p. Superpulse T_p should be shorter than the thermal relaxation time of tissue. The T_r of the superpulse waveform is similarly optimized for tissue cooling between pulses. Incisions are best made with SP, because there are negligible coagulative properties in tissue responding to this mode of laser energy delivery.

The superpulse waveform can also be pulsed. During each macropulse of the SP waveform there are several micropulses of laser energy output. A single superpulse T_p is generally 200 to 300 µsec and repeats at 150 to 250 Hz depending on T_r. A common use of SP in PW mode is to create 25 msec macropulses at 30 Hz of SP micropulses at 200 Hz. This allows a T_r between macropulses of about 8.333 msec to permit a greater degree of tissue cooling.

The top waveform illustrates a series of continuous superpulses, or a macropulse of superpulse micropulses. The lower waveform illustrates a pulsed superpulse in which each macropulse would feature a brief run of constituent micropulses.

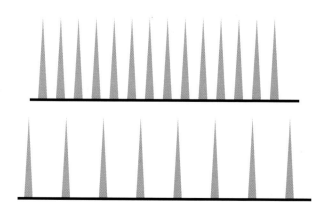

may reach 10^7 to 10^9 watts! Q-switching is produced by cyclically disturbing the standing wave created within the optical resonant cavity while maintaining strong pumping. The result is a short burst of extremely high power at the instant the disturbance is released. Finally, cavity dumping occurs when a large population inversion (photon cascade) is created very quickly and the strongly reinforced beam of laser light is trapped within the resonant cavity. All of the coherent light is then released in a short pulse of high power.

The power that a laser delivers can be controlled by changing the diameter of the beam or the amount of time that the energy is delivered. The circular pattern that laser light produces at its target is referred to as the *spot size*. This is the diameter of the beam at its contact point with the target agent. Most lasers produce a circular spot unless the beam geometry is altered. The spot size can be changed by using focusing tips or lensed focusing hand pieces or by changing the distance between the focusing tip and the target. In contrast, the intensity of a collimated beam is only altered by managing its power. Successful surgical laser use requires an understanding of the relationship between power output and spot size of the beam, distance to the target tissue, the angle of targeting, and length of delivery time.

Chapter 2
Power Density and the Basic Effects of Radiant Energy on Tissue

When discussing different kinds of laser-producing compounds, molecules, or atoms, the type of material closed within the resonant chamber defines the laser identification. The material that is used for the lasing process without being expended is often related to the name of the laser itself, *e.g.*, the CO_2 laser has CO_2 gas as the lasing medium. There are liquid, solid, and gas lasers. It is possible to obtain lasing action from many of these materials, provided their atomic structure is appropriate, as previously discussed, with respect to the ability to repeatedly produce photons without being self-depleting.

All lasers, including medical lasers, are referred to in terms of their wavelength in nanometers (nm), microns (um), or millimeters (mm). Lasers occupy a relatively small portion of the entire electromagnetic spectrum. Photons of this type can be produced from any region of the light spectrum. In most cases the energy requirement costs far exceed the photon output for useable laser energy. But in certain cases the photon-output-to-energy-requirement ratio is efficient enough to allow for the economical and reproducible production of laser energy that can do work on target materials or tissues.

There are currently a significant number of wavelengths available for veterinary clinical use. In fact, many newer devices can be finely dialed in to emit photons at the exact wavelength, amplitude, and frequency that match the particular target source in body tissues to bring about their selective energy uptake with subsequent disruption and vaporization. This intense, pure beam of coherent collimated light follows the basic laws of photon-to-tissue interaction that is referred to as photobiology. Thus, a consistent and reproducible effect can be predicted and induced to provide a variety of treatment options.

There are also ways to enhance, alter, or modify the wavelengths from standard lasers. Certain crystal structure forms, called *nonlinear asymmetric crystals*, can take the laser and, through an interaction of these photons with the crystal lattice structure, generate laser light with twice the frequency (half the wavelength) of the originating laser wavelength. This is known as *frequency doubling* or *harmonic generation*. By using these crystals in conjunction with lasers, it is possible to significantly alter the wavelength by double, triple, or quadruple the wavelengths from the primary laser source. It is also possible to use one laser to excite another and, by using liquid dyes that can go into many different meta-stable states, obtain a whole variety of different wavelengths from a single laser device. This is very important when considering that varying wavelengths of laser energy interact in specific and finite ways with target materials or tissues based on target tissue component uptake of the laser energy.

Power Density

The intensity of a laser beam is best described using the extremely important concept of *power density*. Power density is measured as the radiant power striking a target per unit area of cross-section of a laser light beam. That power, P, is described as the amount of energy delivered per unit of time. Power density, P_o, is generally stated in units of W/cm^2.

$$P = e / t$$

$$P_o = P / A$$

Power density is directly proportional to the power (in watts) that a laser can deliver, and inversely proportional to the surface area (in cm^2) that the beam strikes to do work.

The fundamental power density profile of a laser beam used in veterinary surgery is the Gaussian, or TEM_{00} mode. This geometric pattern is ideal because it can be focused to a very small effective diameter on a target. The smallest possible effective diameter at the focal point of a laser beam is

$$d_{min} = 2f\lambda/(\pi r)$$

where *r* is the radius of the beam where it enters the lens or focusing tip having focal length, *f*, through which laser light of wavelength λ will converge. The CO_2 laser has a wavelength of 10.6 μm. When this invisible light passes through a 1.5mm diameter aperture, the smallest effective diameter that can be produced by focusing through a tip having a focal length of 3mm is 27 microns—just over two wavelengths. For practical use, though, the smallest diameter laser beam that a focusing tip will produce is equal to the size of its opening, *i.e.*, 0.3mm.

The effective diameter of a laser beam, d_e, is conveniently described as the diameter of a concentric circle perpendicular to the axis of beam propagation that contains 86.5% of the total power of the laser beam, as noted in Chapter 1. Note that peak power exists only at the axis, and falls exponentially toward zero away from the axis. The effective diameter of a laser beam is a convenient value to use when discussing spot size or any other parameter regarding the power density of a laser beam.

Simply increasing or decreasing the power delivered through any given constant effective diameter can influence power density, and that change will be strictly linear. For example, if 8 watts (power) are delivered to a circular spot that is 0.8mm diameter, the power density is approximately 1280 W/cm^2, from the following calculation:

$$P_o = P/\pi r = (8 \text{ W} \times 4)/ \pi(0.08 \text{ cm})^2$$

The power density can be increased to 2,560 W/cm^2 by increasing power to 16 watts, and decreased to 640 W/cm^2 by decreasing power to 4 watts. Thus, doubling the power will double the power density if the effective diameter remains constant. Likewise, reducing the power by a factor of one-third will also reduce the power density one-third. This is a strictly linear relationship.

More dramatic effects in power density changes are observed by altering the diameter of the delivery of that beam, and those changes obey an inverse square law.

Assuming a circular spot size and constant power delivered, the change in power density will change with the inverse square of the effective diameter of the beam. For example, if 10W are applied through effective diameters of 1.4mm, 0.8mm, 0.4mm, and 0.3mm, the corresponding power densities would be 648 W/cm^2, 1,984 W/cm^2, 7,938 W/cm^2, 14,111 W/cm^2. Note that by doubling the effective diameter from 0.4mm to 0.8mm the power density is diminished by one-fourth and that power density quadruples by using an effective diameter that is comparatively one-half as wide. Likewise, the difference in power density changes by a factor of approximately 25 when comparing the effective diameters of 0.3mm and 1.4mm. (Figure 2-1)

The average power density, in W/cm^2, of an unfocused collimated beam of light, or light that has passed through a cylindrical quartz fiber, is given by the total beam power divided by the cross sectional area of the beam:

$$P_o = P/\pi r^2 = 127.3\, P_o / (d_e \text{ in mm})^2$$

This approximation does not apply for focused beams. Normally a focused beam will converge from the distal end of its delivery system to a finite focal point, then diverge from this focal point to infinite expansion. This divergence can be used for the surgeon's benefit if it is understood that changing the distance from the target will change the power density of the beam at the point of tissue contact. For collimated beams, changing the distance from the target has no influence on power density at the tissue target. (Figure 2-2)

The focal distance, *f*, of a typical CO_2 laser-focusing tip is 2 mm from its aperture. This means the power density of the beam will be highest near this point, and lower power densities will be found either proximal or distal to this focal point. In actuality this system prevents a perfect focal point, but there is a focal area in the range of 1 mm to 3 mm from the opening, but for simplicity, we will describe the focal distance as 2 mm. A circular area at the focal point having diameter d_e will possess

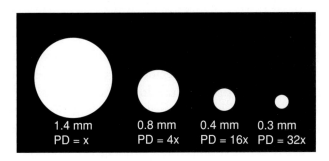

Figure 2-1 The power density of a focused laser beam is dramatically changed by altering its effective diameter. For approximately circular areas, changes in power density obey an inverse square law according to changes in spot size diameter. Reducing the diameter of the spot by 50% increases the power density fourfold; and likewise, doubling the diameter of the spot diminishes power density to one-fourth of the original.

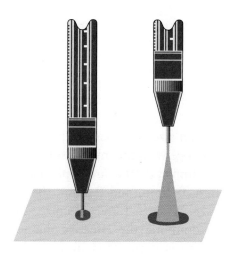

Figure 2-2 A focused laser beam has a focal area located 1 mm to 3 mm from the aperture of a focusing tip. The laser beam will diverge beyond that focal area. Observe that the spot diameter will increase as the handpiece and focusing tip are separated a greater distance from the target. This increase in diameter will reduce the delivered power density. Also note that the angle of divergence will differ among focusing tips. Widely divergent angles will cause a much greater and much faster reduction in power density with any changes in distance to the target from the focal area. This does not apply for collimated beams, in which case the power density does not change at all with any change in distance from the aperture to the target.

An experienced surgeon can use the ability to change power density with distance when it is desirable to rapidly change surgical technique from ablation at high power density to coagulation at lower power density. Simply increasing the distance from the laser tip to the target will achieve this goal. It is important to not touch the tissue with a focusing tip because the laser beam is converging from the tip opening down to the focal area, and also to avoid clogging the aperture.

power density P_o. The spot size on a plane perpendicular to the beam axis at a focal distance from the focal point will have a diameter that varies with the angle of divergence, θ, from the focusing tip. Smaller size focusing tips will have higher divergent angles and larger size focusing tips will have smaller angles of divergence. The diameter of that spot is approximately calculated from:

$$d_e = f \sin \theta$$

The power density at this point is similarly approximated by:

$$P_o = 4P/(\pi f^2 \sin^2 \theta)$$

Note that power density is inversely related to the square of the focal distance, f, and inversely related to the square of the sine of the angle of divergence. For focusing tips having the same focal length, f, the change in spot size produced at a given distance from the focal point will be greater if the divergent angle, θ, is larger. Likewise, a tip having a smaller divergent angle will have smaller changes in spot size at a given distance from the focal area. Simply moving the focusing tip, or the end of the fiber, toward or away from the target will produce significant alterations in power density at the target tissue. Doubling the distance from the focal point will reduce power density by more than one-fourth. Note that this does not always apply when changing the target area to a location proximal to the focal area. Contacting the tissues with a focused tip, or using a focusing tip as a surgical probe, will certainly produce disastrous results due to defocusing effects on the tissue and from thermal injury through alteration in tissue interaction, as will be discussed. Thus, smaller focusing tips can produce higher power density, but moving away from the target causes precipitous drops in power density that may be harmful or ineffectual. Larger focusing tips produce lower power densities, but do not cause rapid fluctuations in power density as a result of distance from the focal area. Optically focused hand pieces can produce the same effect. These often have a metal guide to provide approximate location to the target tissue of average optimal focal distance for the converging beam to be at its maximum focus.

To deliver the full benefit of the power to a surgical site, the laser beam should be focused to its optimal focal diameter at the target tissue and perpendicular to it (this concept is used repeatedly to produce optimal results, as seen in the Case Studies section). Any deviation from optimal position will cause a loss of power applied to the tissue and potentially undesirable effects, as will be discussed in Chapter 3. For a perfectly normal beam, the incident power density, P_i, is equal to the power density delivered to the target, P_d. However, much power can be lost (Figure 2-3) if the surgeon applies the laser beam at an angle θ deviated from normal, such that,

$$P_o = P_i \sin \theta.$$

Other important aspects of power density changes to the target tissue will occur, resulting from some light reflected at the surgical surface, and some will be transmitted through the surface to exert its effect on tissue, as will be discussed in Chapters 3 and 4.

Basic Effects of Radiant Energy on Tissue

Ideally, a laser surgeon incises, vaporizes, or cuts tissue and uses adequate power density applied at the optimal focal area of the beam, and directs that beam perpendicular to the tissue to achieve the surgical precision that a laser offers for that target tissue. Other effects are possible, *i.e.*, defocusing the beam by moving farther away from the target and thus decreasing power density by increasing the spot size, and/or directing the beam at an angle to tissue, thus causing a decrease in power density as described previously. The effect of using below-vaporization-threshold-power density is, depending on how far below threshold the power density is, coagulation, collagen contraction, protein denaturation, and heating of tissue, which will be discussed. Ablation of tissue can be a useful application of a surgical laser, but if not controlled properly, an inexperienced surgeon may produce morbid consequences to the target tissue. It is important for

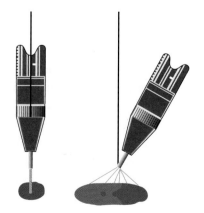

Figure 2-3 A laser beam directed perpendicular (normal) to the target will produce the greatest degree of interaction. Any deviation from normal by an angle will cause lower power densities at the target due to distortion of the spot geometry. Note that the resulting power density is also non-uniform: the proximal area has increased fluence, and the distal area has decreased fluence.

any laser surgeon to understand the surgical significance of power density and how its diversity produces various tissue effects before beginning to use a laser for therapeutic or surgical intervention.

As previously discussed, the varieties of surgical lasers presently available produce different wavelengths of light depending, on their medium. The target tissue composition and the laser wavelength determine how the tissue reacts upon illumination. Laser light focused on tissue can causes five different optical phenomena at the tissue/laser interface. It may be reflected, refracted, transmitted, absorbed, or scattered. Laser light is converted to other forms of energy when absorbed within the target tissue. In order of increasing magnitude of energy, these laser-tissue interactions are classified as *photochemical, photothermal,* or *photoplasmolytic,* depending on whether the absorbed laser energy is converted to chemical, thermal, or mechanical-acoustic energy.

Photochemical reactions occur when laser light is absorbed and converted into chemical energy. This energy directly breaks complex organic biochemical bonds, resulting in tissue destruction or alteration. Excimer lasers, or lasers whose wavelengths are very short in the ultraviolet range, are generally used for *photochemolysis*. Photodynamic therapy, or PDT, is achieved by photochemolysis using a photosensitizer, a light-reactive target drug that can be administered intravenously, orally, topically, or intralesionally. The photosensitizer should optimally localize at the target tissue site by concentrating within its blood supply or tissue fluid component. When a laser wavelength of matching frequency uptake interacts with the photosensitizer the laser-activated photosensitizer initiates the destruction of the chemically labeled tissue. This typically occurs by biochemical bond disruption or thermal effect, destabilizing the cell membrane.

Photothermolysis occurs when the energy of laser light is converted to heat at the target tissue interface, causing the temperature of the target tissue to rise rapidly. Water, hemoglobin, melanin, and some proteins within the target tissue absorb varying wavelengths of laser light, resulting in tissue heating. These are the component agents for laser/tissue interaction. As the temperature of tissue heats to of 42° to 60° C, hyperthermia may contract, constrict, or destroy blood vessels, resulting in tissue hypoxia and cell death. As tissue temperatures increase to 60° to 100° C, coagulation occurs, collagen contracts, proteins are denatured, and irreversible tissue damage occurs concomitantly with dehydration and/or desiccation at a cellular level. As the tissue is superheated above 100° C, vaporization occurs via almost instantaneous boiling of intracellular water and solid tissue is converted to gaseous vapor and a smoke plume. The superheating of tissue and vaporization leads to carbonization remnant formation of non-fluid cellular components known as char. This black char readily absorbs laser energy at any wavelength. Continued lasing of char such as by repeated passes over a specific area without char removal furthers the absorption of laser energy without the potential for vaporization, and thermal energy continues to accumulate within the tissues in the form of radiant heat. The thermal energy is conducted to the surrounding tissues rapidly but below vaporization threshold, resulting in hyperthermia and collateral tissue damage. The remaining carbon char also acts as a foreign substance, creating the potential for increased inflammation. Furthermore, char can act as an inert layer under which bacteria can multiply and create incision site infection and an inflammatory response. The combination of thermal injury and foreign material in a surgical site can cause coagulative necrosis and delayed wound healing with a strong potential for infection and wound dehiscence.

Photopyrolytic laser-tissue interaction results in tissue coagulation. This process occurs when tissues reach temperatures between 60° and 100° C as a result of the absorption of laser energy at the target tissue that is transformed into heat. The classic coagulative laser uses Nd:YAG or a diode as the lasing medium in contact mode. The laser energy is converted to heat at the wave guide tip and applied to the target tissue. More commonly, though, if a surgeon desires to incise or cut tissue *via* vaporization, the laser beam must have enough power density to cause the tissues to reach 100° C very rapidly (Figure 2-4).

Photovaporolysis is the process wherein the histologic water is rapidly flashed over to steam. This rapidly expands and ruptures the relatively weak cell membranes and disrupts the normal tissue structure. A plume of desiccated carbonaceous material and water vapor is ejected away from the surgery site. Far less conduction of heat (less than 0.1%) is distributed to surrounding tissues as compared to photopyrolysis. The two most commonly used lasers in soft tissue surgery are either the Er:YAG or CO_2 because of their strong photovaporolytic effects. Diode lasers in contact mode can also produce a photovaporolytic effect to pigmented tissues, but only if the power density is high.

Mechanical-acoustic disruption can be achieved by a phenomenon called *photoplasmolysis*. This occurs when rapidly pulsed laser light is converted to acoustical energy that forms a target-tissue-disrupting shock wave at the leading edge of the tissue/laser interface. The laser beam needs to be of exceedingly high power density such that the light waves are strong enough to ionize the atoms in the tissue and form a *plasma*. In this physical case, a plasma is a confined area of an exceedingly hot gas

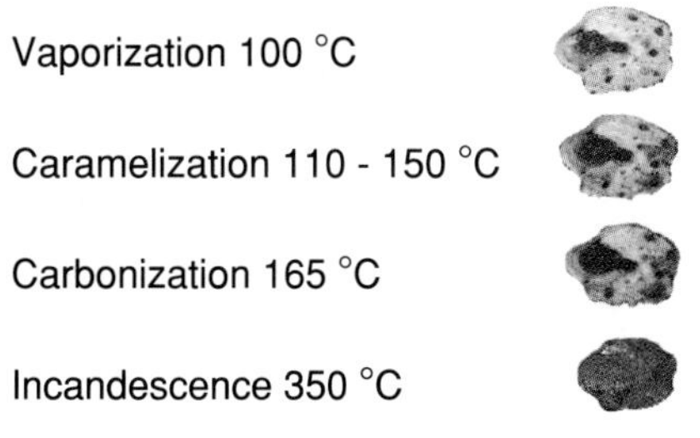

**The Effects of
Thermal Energy Accumulation**

Denaturation 55 - 60 °C

Coagulation 60 - 80 °C

Vacuolization 80 - 95 °C

Vaporization 100 °C

Caramelization 110 - 150 °C

Carbonization 165 °C

Incandescence 350 °C

Figure 2-4 The process of photothermolysis is irreversible. It is caused by the absorption of light energy and its transformation to heat energy that accumulates within tissue. Slow rates of thermal energy accumulation generally cause coagulative necrosis and conduction of heat by radiation through tissue. Extremely high rates of thermal energy accumulation cause instantaneous vaporization and ablation of tissue without thermal conduction.

The progressive heating of an egg until it is cooked and then burned shows this process on a large scale. The actual events of photothermolysis occur at the cellular/tissue level within μsec to msec.

(>3,000° C) consisting of equal concentrations of free electrons and positive ions. A plasma ball is a strong absorber of all wavelengths of light. Once the plasma is formed at the tissue it absorbs all incoming laser light and expands rapidly. This expanding, leading plasma wave front causes a shock wave and mechanical disruption of tissue. Only ultra-short-pulsed lasers are capable of photoplasmolysis due to the high power density ($> 10^{10}$ W/cm^2) that is required for its production. A good example of this is canine lithotripsy, which is performed with a Ho:YAG laser.

For any wavelength that is absorbed by water there is a threshold of power density below which the water in the target tissue cannot be vaporized by a laser beam. This threshold is lower for wavelengths that are strongly absorbed by water, *e.g.*, 2,900 nm for Er:YAG or 10,600 nm for CO$_2$. This threshold is also highest for those wavelengths that are poorly absorbed, *e.g.*, visible light lasers 400 nm to 700 nm. When the rate of heat dissipation from the tissues exceeds the rate of heat deposition within the tissues, the water will either be warmed or heated and neither boiled nor vaporized. At wavelengths that scatter significantly within tissue, the net effect will be photopyrolysis, which can be used for controlled coagulation but generally is not very efficient for incising or cutting. Wavelengths that are highly absorbed by water will generally be attenuated rapidly at the surface of tissues, allowing for shallow penetration depths. These lasers are highly efficient for cutting and incising yet do not cause sufficient collateral heating to provide coagulation of vessels greater than 0.6 mm in diameter.

If a surgeon desires to coagulate tissue without vaporizing it, the power density of the beam must not exceed the threshold of vaporization at that wavelength. The wavelength also should be poorly absorbed by histologic water and be scattered within the tissue, causing the conversion of laser energy to thermal energy and a slow increase in the temperature of the tissue. On the other hand, if a surgeon desires to precisely incise or cut tissue with minimal heating of surrounding tissues, the power density of the beam should far exceed the threshold of vaporization at that wavelength. The wavelength should be highly absorbed by water so that the light is attenuated rapidly as well. This causes rapid vaporization of tissue with minimal thermal conduction, but the ability to coagulate tissue is dramatically limited. There are conditions whereby a wavelength that causes coagulation can be used to cut, and likewise, there are conditions whereby a wavelength that causes vaporization can be used to coagulate. To the extent that one wavelength can vaporize tissue, it loses the ability to coagulate. Alternatively, wavelengths that produce good coagulation are generally poorly ablative. (Figures 2-5 and 2-6)

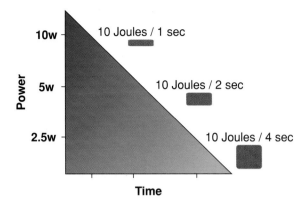

Figure 2-5 The units in this representation of the ablation threshold have been simplified for clarity. Ten watts of power can be produced by delivering 10J in 1 second but this is unrealistic. Assuming 10W are passed through a 0.4 mm diameter focusing tip, this is sufficient power density to exceed the ablation threshold, and power below this would cause coagulation but not ablation.

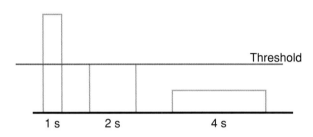

Figure 2-6 Note that although fluence is equal in each of these three examples, the ablation threshold can be exceeded only when sufficient fluence is delivered in a short period of time. Excess fluence beyond the ablation threshold is absorbed by tissue at greater penetration depths. Subthreshold fluence causes accumulation of heat and coagulative necrosis of tissue.

Chapter 3
Fundamentals of Laser-Tissue Interactions

Four basic interactions can take place when laser energy interacts with a target material or tissue: reflection, scatter, or transmission, or absorption (Figure 3-1). The desired interaction is straightforward (Chapter 2) yet dynamic in its process. The positive thermal effects produced by the absorption of laser energy can provide localized vaporization with a negligible degree of hyperthermia, coagulation, and necrosis. However, reflection, scatter, and transmission may cause uncontrolled effects on the target tissue or adjacent tissue structures.

When laser energy interacts with tissue above the vaporization threshold, the photothermal effect produces a vaporization impact site or laser vaporization crater (Figure 3-2). The tissue that has been vaporized from this region disperses in a plume composed of remnant particles of the tissue and water vapor. Two distinct regions immediately surround the trough. Closest to the vaporization trough region is an area of hyperthermia, cellular coagulation, and necrosis. This zone is created by multiple, variable, and alterable laser energy interactions from the point of laser energy impact. This can be as small as 0.01 mm or as large as 2 to 3 mm. Immediately adjacent to this zone is an area of cellular edema without evidence of alteration in the cellular integrity or collagen denaturation. Thermal relaxation in this region is rapid enough to avoid desiccation or collagen contracture. This allows cellular function and cell membrane integrity to be spared. The milder thermal injury to the tissue in this region may resolve immediately or up to 72 hours later.

The ultimate goal is for the target tissue to absorb the laser energy by adequately controlling reflection, scatter, and transmission. When tissue absorbs the energy of laser light it converts the light into other forms of energy, empowering laser energy to do surgical work on the target tissue. On the other hand, reflection of laser energy can occur when the energy fails to be absorbed and is deflected in the direction from which it came or at an acute angle to its origin. Laser energy can be reflected off of the first surface of interaction; this is sometimes referred to as "heating back." The light also transmits through target tissue to varying penetration depths, depending on the wavelength, and may also experience refraction as the light passes from one medium interface through another. The light can also be scattered within the tissue, because the particulate nature of cytoplasmic contents makes histologic targets neither homogeneous nor isotropic.

This chapter explains these phenomena of laser-tissue interaction and how the choice of wavelength, time of its use, and the physical characteristics of the targeted tissue are interdependent for favorable surgical outcomes. It shows that by knowing the physical characteristics of tissue-laser interaction, a surgeon can selectively use an appropriate wavelength of laser energy for the proper time period to achieve the desired effect without morbid consequences.

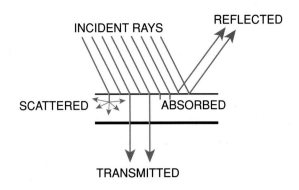

Figure 3-1 The four basic interactions of light at the surface it strikes. A reflective surface does not allow the transmission of light. Light that is transmitted through a medium may be absorbed, and these two properties are inversely related to each other. Particles within a medium may also scatter light. The extent to which these four interactions occur depends upon the medium as well as the wavelength of light.

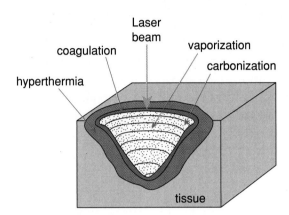

Figure 3-2 A representation of a crater produced in tissue by a burst of laser energy that exceeded ablation threshold. The crater's 3-D geometry is Gaussian, essentially the same shape as the power density profile of the laser beam described in Figure 1-15. The zone of carbonization is the limit of vaporization. Slightly farther away from the center of the crater is the zone of coagulation and thermal necrosis. This zone will eventually die. Farthest from the center is the zone of hyperthermia. Here the temperature of the tissue has slightly increased, but will cool down quickly. Beyond these zones there is no effect. Both the depth of the crater and the diameter of these zones are directly related to power density.

The chapter first examines the negative effects of laser energy—why the effects occur, their potential results, and how to prevent them. Those discussions are followed by an in-depth look at the desirable laser-tissue interaction, absorption.

Reflection

The reflection of light from a surface is a generally well-understood concept. The path of a ray of light is altered by a reflective surface such that the angle of incidence is equal to the angle of reflection. Laser light will reflect to varying degrees at biological surface interfaces depending on the tissue and the wavelength. In biological systems, there may also be an effect from the backscattering of light as it strikes a particulate medium. Notwithstanding basic optical physics, if the angle of incidence is 0°, some light will be reflected back to its source; and if the angle of incidence is 90°, the light will not change its course. A basic parameter of reflective surfaces is the *reflectance* or the ratio of the reflected light intensity to the incident light intensity. In general, it is desirable for an optical mirror to have a reflectance greater than 97%.

$$R = P_r / P_i$$

The reflectance of biological tissue is based upon the efficiency of power density conservation at the target surface, and is strongly dependent on wavelength. There is a pronounced reflectance of wavelengths in the range of 400 nm to 1,500 nm. Laser light is also reflected away much more by lightly colored (unpigmented) skin. Erythrocytes, brain tissue, cartilage, muscle, and liver also reflect laser light more significantly at these wavelengths. Note that reflectance is absent below 300 nm and above 2,000nm. Therefore, a CO_2 laser will not reflect its light because the wavelength of 10.6 μm is well outside of this range. In strong contrast, the power delivered by a Nd:YAG laser at 1,064 nm is diminished in half at the target surface due to target surface reflection, especially if the target is light skin or a bloody field. The most profound effect of the loss of power density due to reflection at the first surface is the reduction of the laser's ability to impart surgical work due to loss of fluence below the target surface.

Light will transmit through a fluid medium according to Beer's law:

$$T = e^{-\epsilon bc}$$

or

$$A = \epsilon bc$$

where *T* is the percent transmission of light through tissue, *A* is the absorbance, ϵ is the molar absorptivity with units of L mol^{-1} cm^{-1}, *b* is the path length of the beam of light, and *c* is the concentration of the compound in solution. The molar absorptivity is a unique constant for a given substance and is different for each individual substance. The law says that the fraction of light absorbed by equivalent layers of solution is constant. This fundamental physical law of solutions is linear and works very well at ordinary concentrations of solutes, but breaks down at exceedingly high concentrations that are not applicable in biological systems. It also proves that light will be absorbed more by solutions with higher concentrations, and will transmit more through solutions with low concentrations. If all the light passes through a solution without any absorption, then absorbance is zero, and transmittance is 100%. If all the light is absorbed, then transmittance is zero, and absorption is infinite (Figure 3-3). There is a mnemonic device to help you remember Beer's Law: ***The taller the glass, the darker the brew, the less the amount of light transmits through!*** This can also apply to tissue thickness and the volume of target-specific interfaces that laser energy must interact with as it contacts the target tissue.

Scatter and Transmission

Scatter and transmission are two additional problems that can occur during laser-tissue interaction. These are usually less preferable than absorption. The tissue itself can scatter the light, which literally bounces off particles and structures within the tissue and scatters to places where it may be absorbed, creating its own tissue interaction. This can adversely affect surrounding tissue. Furthermore, the light may be transmitted right

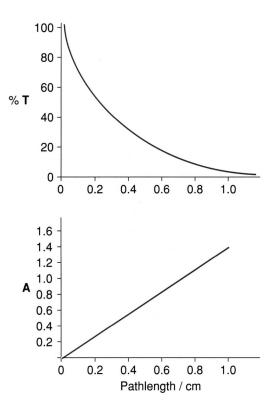

Figure 3-3 Graphical illustration of Beer's law. This shows a direct relationship between absorption of light and the length of the path through which it travels. There also is a logarithmic decrease in the transmission of light with increasing path length.

through the tissue, maintaining its energy with only a minimal effect on the target tissue. This occurs when the light wavelength is not interacted on by an appropriate pigment or absorption medium in the targeted tissue. Since every tissue has reflective, scattering, and transmitting properties, understanding these tissue characteristics is a critical aspect of knowing how the specific form of laser energy you are using will affect the target tissue. Understanding this concept can provide the clinician with the most favorable laser-tissue interaction.

Laser light transmits through tissue to the degree that it has not been reflected, scattered, absorbed, or *refracted*. Refraction of a laser beam occurs when it crosses the interface of two media having different indices of refraction, changing its wavelength, direction, and speed. The speed of light, *c*, is reduced according to the index of refraction of the medium, *n*, such that:

$$v_m = c / n$$

Since the light's frequency does not change, but its speed does, its wavelength must be changed as well as its direction when transmitting between two media of different indices of refraction:

$$\lambda = v_m / f$$

The ray's change in direction is calculated based on its deviation from normal, or an imaginary line drawn perpendicular to the target surface:

$$\sin \theta_1 / \sin \theta_2 = n_2 / n_1$$

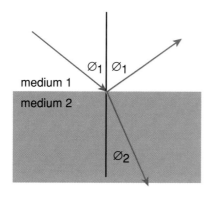

Figure 3-4 A ray of light strikes a reflective/ transmissive interface such as tissue. The angle of incidence, θ, is equal to the angle of reflection. The media have two different indices of refraction. In this example $n_2 > n_1$, and the penetrating beam of light is refracted toward normal and $\theta_2 < \theta_1$.

Note that the angle of deviation from normal will be higher in the medium with a lower refractive index, and media with a higher refractive index will create a smaller deviation. Also note that if $n_2 > n_1$, light travels slower in the medium with a higher index of refraction, the direction of the beam of laser light will be closer to normal and $\theta_2 < \theta_1$, which means the beam may not terminate where the surgeon desires but will fall short of its intended target area (Figure 3-4).

When a light ray interacts with a particle it may change direction without changing its wavelength, and thus is said to scatter. The type and degree of scatter depends on both the incident wavelength and the size of the particle. Scattering of light by particles much smaller than the wavelength of incident light ($< 1/10^{th}\ \lambda$) is known as Rayleigh scattering. Rayleigh scattering is strongly dependent on wavelength and is omnidirectional:

$$P_R = p_o \frac{8\pi^4\ N\ \alpha^2}{\lambda^4\ R^2}\ (1+\cos^2\theta)$$

It is much easier and more practical to describe the effects of Rayleigh scattering of light as strongly inversely proportional to the fourth power of the wavelength being scattered by small particles. Thus, the effect is much stronger for shorter wavelengths:

$$P_R \propto 1/\lambda^4$$

Such scattering of light is equally intense in the forward and backward direction, and half as energetic perpendicular to the original ray. This type of scatter is not important for laser-tissue interaction, but it is of interest in answering the question, "Why is the sky blue"? At 400 nm, the scattering of blue light is 9.4 times as great as that of red light at 700 nm. The strong wavelength dependency of Rayleigh scattering ensures that an observer on the ground will see predominantly blue light well after sunrise or well before sunset, yet predominantly red light is seen during sunrise and sunset since the blue light is strongly scattered away.

When scattering is caused by a particle whose diameter is comparable to or greater than the wavelength of the light, it demonstrates a different type of scattering, named after Mie, the scientist who described it. Mie scattering of light by particles greater than or equal to its wavelength is

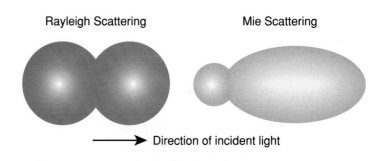

Rayleigh Scattering   Mie Scattering

→ Direction of incident light

Figure 3-5 Rayleigh scattering of light by very small particles is strongly dependant on the wavelength of incident light and is bilobed/omnidirectional. Shorter wavelengths of light are scattered to a much greater degree by particles < 10% of wavelength. Mie scattering of light occurs when an incident ray strikes a particle greater than or equal to wavelength. It is predominantly forward scatter and not as dependant on wavelength as Rayleigh scatter.

more dependent on particle size than wavelength of light (Figures 3-5 and 3-6). This predominantly forward-directed lobular scattering produces a sharper, more intense pattern for larger particles. Mie scattering explains why clouds appear bright white on a sunny day. Mie scattering of light within a fog of water vapor also demonstrates randomly diffused radiant flux, or the appearance of light being equally bright and coming from all directions. Mie scattering is far less dependent on wavelength than Rayleigh scattering, and varies inversely proportionally to the square root of the wavelength:

$$P_M \alpha \; 1/\sqrt{\lambda}$$

Because many histologic micro-architectural structures and cytologic organelles are significantly larger than the wavelengths of laser light, especially lasers in the range between 600 nm and 2,200 nm, diode laser surgeons must be very concerned about Mie scattering within tissues. At higher wavelengths, such as 10.6 µm, scattering is less of a concern. For the laser surgeon, the most important result of scattering is the spatial redistribution of radiant power density from what would otherwise be a coherent collimated monochromatic beam of light into the surrounding tissue. Once the light is dispersed throughout a volume of tissue, it is absorbed and attenuated.

Figure 3-6 Clouds are brightly white when observed in front of the sun due to Mie scattering. Since blue light has a shorter wavelength than red light, it is Rayleigh scattered to a greater degree, which explains why the sky may appear blue after sunset or before sunrise.

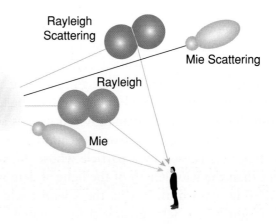

Rayleigh Scattering   Mie Scattering

Rayleigh

Mie

Absorption

The process of absorption of laser energy by a tissue is the key to effective laser-to-tissue interaction. When photons enter the tissue, those that are not reflected, scattered, or transmitted are absorbed. Maximizing the absorption effect and minimizing other effects produces the most consistent, reproducible lasing results for the clinician. The photonic energy is transferred to other molecules or groups of atoms within the tissue that then causes them to be altered or vaporized as previously discussed. Once this photonic energy is absorbed, it transfers its energy potential to the target tissue, thus inducing a change in that tissue. This is really the key to producing the different tissue changes needed during clinical or surgical treatment using laser energy.

From lowest level to highest level of absorption, these conversion processes occur as follows: 1) elevating molecules to higher energy states, 2) effecting stored chemical energy, 3) fluorescence, or the re-radiation of energy at a lower energy level with inherent energy loss, 4) transformation into kinetic energy as heat or vibrations, and 5) creation of plasma, a superheated ionized gas.

For surgical purposes, only the conversion of radiant energy to kinetic energy is useful. Excitation, chemical potential energy, and fluorescence all have their place in science but may not be immediately practical to the general veterinary surgeon. As discussed in Chapter 2, a surgical laser heats intracellular components very rapidly to produce the desired vaporization effect. This occurs due to the tissue's rapid absorption of radiant energy, or photothermolysis.

Photoplasmolysis occurs when extremely high power densities ($>10^9$ W/cm^2) target tissues during extremely short periods of time (picoseconds to nanoseconds). When tissues are heated to the point of incandescence, the surrounding air becomes ionized and forms a small sphere of plasma. This plasma is a strong absorber of all laser wavelengths and absorbs the energy of the laser beam. The energy absorption causes a rapid expansion of the sphere and creates a shock wave that can disrupt tissue and shatter hard substances, *e.g.*, calculi. Many laser surgeons have reported that they have seen this incandescence as a white spark at the tissue, and heard the shockwave as a snapping sound at the surface.

As the tissue absorbs laser energy there will be exponentially less energy from the initial beam as it travels deeper into the tissue. That is, a laser beam loses a constant fraction of its intensity per equal unit of distance traveled. This phenomenon is called *attenuation* and is extremely important to relate to surgical tissue handling. The power density of a laser beam is attenuated within tissue according to Bouger's law (which is very similar to Beer's law):

$$p_z = p_o\, e^{-Az}$$

where p_z is the power density at depth z beyond the tissue surface (note: also take into account the effects of reflection and non-normal incidence of the light ray to calculate p_o), and A is the attenuation coefficient. Since both *absorption*, α, and *scattering*, σ, contribute to the attenuation of a light ray traveling through tissue, the attenuation coefficient is defined as:

$$A = \alpha + \sigma$$

The absorption coefficient of a particular medium depends on the targeted tissue as well as the wavelength of laser light. The scattering coefficient, however, is primarily depends on wavelength. Scattering coefficients are higher at shorter wavelengths. Mie scattering is more important than Rayleigh scattering within tissues, and this scatter is primarily forward and caused by interaction of light with larger particles. Mie scattering of light within tissues and reflection of light away from tissues is most significant in the range between 600 nm and 2,200 nm.

The absorption of light strongly depends on the tissue's physical characteristics. The noteworthy components of living tissue that absorb light are water, pigments, lipids, hemoglobin, oxyhemoglobin, and carbon. Since the surgeon is keenly aware of the constituents of target tissue before using any laser for surgery, the choice of wavelength for a given procedure is dictated by that tissue's absorption component characteristics. This is important because an improperly chosen wavelength produces undesired effects and untoward surgical outcomes, yet an appropriately chosen wavelength which has excellent absorption in the surgical tissue is a useful surgical tool in the hands of a qualified surgeon.

There are significant differences between the amount of absorption of photonic energy by water or pigments within tissue. The surgeon may be able to cause selective destruction of the target tissue simply by choosing the appropriate laser wavelength for the operation, thereby sparing surrounding tissue or eliminating peripheral heat transfer. As will be discussed later, the choice of laser for soft tissue surgery should be based on the predominant tissue component and the desired surgical effect (Figure 3-7).

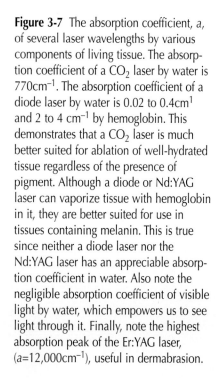

Figure 3-7 The absorption coefficient, *a*, of several laser wavelengths by various components of living tissue. The absorption coefficient of a CO_2 laser by water is $770 cm^{-1}$. The absorption coefficient of a diode laser by water is 0.02 to $0.4 cm^{1}$ and 2 to $4 cm^{-1}$ by hemoglobin. This demonstrates that a CO_2 laser is much better suited for ablation of well-hydrated tissue regardless of the presence of pigment. Although a diode or Nd:YAG laser can vaporize tissue with hemoglobin in it, they are better suited for use in tissues containing melanin. This is true since neither a diode laser nor the Nd:YAG laser has an appreciable absorption coefficient in water. Also note the negligible absorption coefficient of visible light by water, which empowers us to see light through it. Finally, note the highest absorption peak of the Er:YAG laser, ($a=12,000 cm^{-1}$), useful in dermabrasion.

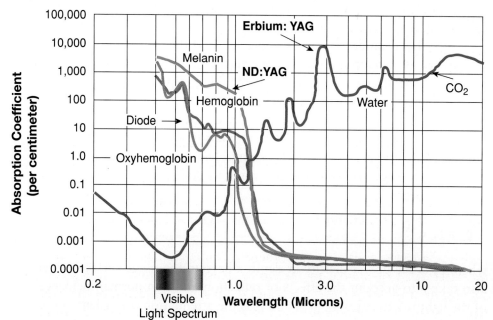

Water is the most abundant substance within tissue and is a strong absorber of light in the near-infrared and ultraviolet wavelengths, but has highest absorption at mid-infrared wavelengths. There is negligible absorption of visible light by water. Water absorbs light maximally at 2,940 nm, the characteristic wavelength of the Erbium:YAG laser. There is also extremely high absorption of light at 10,600 nm, the wavelength produced by a CO_2 laser. Also note that visible light is negligibly absorbed by water, and the near infrared light of the Nd:YAG laser at 1,064 nm is only moderately absorbed by water. Diode laser light produced between 600 nm and 980 nm is poorly absorbed by water, and that absorption increases slightly as the wavelength increases within that range. Adipose tissue, fats, and lipids often make up a significant portion of a surgical field and absorb light in a similar pattern to water absorption of photonic energy.

Pigments in tissue are also important absorbers of light. They are more highly absorbed in the visible and very-near infrared light wavelength range. Melanin, hemoglobin, and oxyhemoglobin are the most important histologic pigments with respect to this effect; however, other organic molecules such as bilirubin and xanthophyll play a role as well. Melanin is the strongest absorber of light in the visible and near infrared range. Hemoglobin and oxyhemoglobin are also both good absorbers of light in the visible range, but not as effective as melanin. The absorption of light by pigments is highest and almost equal toward the blue and ultraviolet end of the spectrum. These absorption coefficients tend to decrease and show greater disparity as the wavelength increases toward red and near-infrared. Also note that as wavelength increases beyond 1,064 nm (Nd:YAG laser), the absorption coefficient very quickly becomes negligible. These factors can play an important role in laser wavelength selection for specific therapeutic or surgical procedures.

Carbon or char (Chapter 2), which is the end-stage product of prolonged thermal change to tissue, is a strong absorber of light at all wavelengths. Irradiating char will cause its temperature to rise quickly like "a kettle on a stove," and thus cause heating of surrounding tissues. Char can be rapidly heated to such high temperatures that the elemental carbon may incandesce, a phenomenon known as "sparking." As discussed previously, when carbon is heated to temperatures near 3,000°C, the surrounding air becomes an ionized gas, or plasma ball, approximately the diameter of the laser spot size. This ball of plasma is also an extremely good absorber of all light wavelengths. When plasma absorbs incoming laser energy it rapidly expands and creates an audible "snap" from the shock wave it creates. This is generally considered undesirable in soft tissue surgery. It can significantly enlarge peripheral thermal tissue heating. Yet in applications such as lithotripsy using a tunable dye laser or Ho:YAG, this is the intentional effect because it produces a "shock wave" of energy, disrupting the stones at intermolecular bonds.

As radiant energy is absorbed, there is exponentially less power from the laser beam available to do work. This attenuation requires consideration of the *extinction depth* and the penetration depth of the light within tissue. The extinction depth is arbitrarily defined as the depth at which the power density is reduced to 1% of the power density at the tissue surface:

$$P_e = 0.01 \ (P_o)$$

and

$$z_e = 4.605/A$$

where z_e is the depth for 99% attenuation. The *penetration depth* is the distance from the tissue surface at which point the laser beam still possesses enough residual power density to produce thermal effects. The extinction depth and the penetration depth are both functions of wavelength and tissue type, but most importantly, the total power density. That is, the extinction depth will always remain constant, but the penetration depth varies proportionally to initial power density. The required thermal effects needed for laser tissue treatment will occur only when the initial power density is high enough. These effects will continue to occur at depths proportional to initial power density and will diminish exponentially by attenuation until the penetration depth has been reached. Varying wavelengths of light penetrate tissue differently. Subthreshold power densities will neither produce thermal effects nor achieve any significant penetration. These differences in absorption of light within tissue help the surgeon choose which wavelength to use for a given purpose.

The choice of a specific laser wavelength for coagulating, vaporizing, or incising tissue then depends on the anticipated laser-tissue interaction. The most important aspects of the behavior of the transmitted light for surgical use are its scatter, transmission, and absorption by the components of the targeted tissue. The scattering and absorption of light by the tissue depends on both the wavelength of light and the tissue itself. It is important to reiterate that the scattering coefficient of tissue, σ, is highest at short wavelengths, and is generally strongest between 600 nm and 2,200 nm. Absorption of light by water and fat in tissue is generally strongest at wavelengths greater than 2,200 nm, and the absorption of light by histologic pigments is predominant between 400 nm and 1,100 nm.

Laser Selection

Lasers that produce wavelengths that are predominantly absorbed by tissue but experience little or no scatter make exceptional incisive tissue vaporizers, but poor coagulators. These lasers generally produce wavelengths greater than 2,500 nm. Because this light is strongly absorbed by tissue, the extinction depth is very shallow, typically less than 1 mm. This is a great advantage for minimizing peripheral or deeper tissue interactions. These lasers are most appropriate for precise surgery due to minimal thermal damage to tissue beyond the effective diameter of the laser beam at appropriate power densities. Classic examples of these "what you see is what you get" (WYSIWYG) lasers are the CO_2 at 10,600 nm and the Erbium:YAG at 2,940 nm. Remember, these are the two peak water absorption coefficients. These ablative WYSIWYG lasers are poor tissue coagulators because their light does not scatter within the target tissue enough to contract blood vessel endothelial linings, but is strongly absorbed and attenuated to extinction within a shallow penetration depth of the tissue surface. 99.2% of the heat that is created is generally ejected out of the vaporization crater as a plume of remnant tissue and water vapor. Only a small amount of residual thermal energy is available for inefficient thermal conduction by surrounding living tissue. These laser wavelengths have short thermal relaxation times. This is a great advantage for the general veterinary surgeon in minimizing unwanted thermal tissue events.

Lasers that produce more coagulating effects are those whose wavelengths are scattered significantly more than they are absorbed by tissue, or are absorbed by multiple tissue components. The pattern of effect within tissue is generally dictated by Mie scattering: predominantly forward, but having concentric half-ovoid isothermal zones of effect surrounding a deep central focus. Every point within this illuminated volume thus acts as a source of heat and causes thermal damage. Increasing the period of time that tissue is targeted will cause these zones of thermal coagulation to become larger, as well. Typically, lasers with wavelengths between 600 nm and 1,400 nm are good tissue coagulators because of the increased tissue that become thermally damaged. Diode lasers (600 nm to 900 nm) and the Nd:YAG laser at 1,064 nm are the classic dissection, coagulative tool. Sometimes they are referred to as "what you don't see can hurt you" (WYDSCHY) because the effects of tissue coagulation and peripheral thermal injury may not be immediately evident. The thermal effects created at a distance from the targeted area may slowly become evident much later on. Furthermore, because of the high amount of scattering within tissue at these wavelengths, it may be difficult to predict both the width and depth of the zone of necrosis or reformation due to thermal coagulation. Depending on the power and time WYDSCHY laser energy is applied, there can be an area affected 5 mm to 10 mm beyond the intended site, and this may occur several hours or even several days following the procedure. This can be desirable when gross tissue ablation is required, due to poorly defined malignant masses, but not when precise delicate tissue handling is required.

There is no single wavelength produced by a laser that will optimally perform every kind of surgical procedure. For precisely incising tissue with minimal thermal necrosis, a WYSIWYG laser such as the CO_2 is ideal. However, if gross ablation of tissue is required, especially if it is pigmented or highly vascular, the experienced veterinary laser surgeon can use a WYDSCHY laser. This is especially true with the diode or Nd:YAG wavelength lasers. There will be some level of collateral thermal necrosis with a CO_2 laser, and conversely a diode or Nd:YAG laser will also incise tissue. It is up to the veterinary laser surgeon to properly understand the equipment-tissue interaction to achieve the desired effect.

As previously discussed, relating to the physics of power density, lasers with more precise vaporization coefficients can be manipulated by defocusing a beam of laser light of wavelength 10,600 nm, causing the spot size to increase and diminish the power density. Lowering the power density in this way will cause more coagulative effects within the tissue solely due to the accumulation of heat via increased scatter and its thermal effects. Because this wavelength does not scatter very well within tissue and is rapidly attenuated, the extent of tissue coagulation is limited. In an opposite example, a typically coagulative wavelength can be used to incise tissue that has a high pigment component. When using the Nd:YAG laser in melanin-rich tissue, or using a diode laser in a vascular field, the rapid and intense absorption of energy by these pigments (and to a lesser extent, water) can cause such rapidly elevated tissue temperatures that the vaporization threshold is exceeded. Vaporization can thus occur with a WYD-SCHY laser, making it behave like a WYSIWYG laser for cutting and excising. Still, peripheral thermal effects will be greater due to the increased scatter of these wavelengths. Likewise, when a WYSIWYG laser is defocused or targeted onto char, it will behave like a WYDSCHY laser and cause coagulation and thermal necrosis.

A veterinary laser surgeon must carefully plan the procedure to achieve the desirable outcome of the patient's safety. The choice of laser must be selected for the intended surgical purpose depending on the tissue characteristics. The surgeon must also decide if the procedure requires cutting, ablation, or coagulation. Non-pigmented tissue will behave very differently than heavily pigmented tissue when a diode or Nd:YAG laser is used. In the same way, fatty or hydrated tissue will behave very differently than bone or desiccated tissue when a CO_2 laser is used. Finally, the choice of laser may also be dictated by the mode of delivery. Depending on the surgical area, diverse delivery systems will be employed to permit using the laser as a surgical tool (Chapter 5).

Key for the clinician is an understanding of where and how this work is produced and how its resultant byproducts are dissipated. Normally, we think of lasers as producing heat. Many of the clinical procedures for which lasers are used involve the production of some kind of local thermal effect. This thermal energy transfer actually provides the effect on the target tissue to alter it or cause its vaporization. The important aspect of using laser energy to produce a tissue effect is to remember that when photons are absorbed, the absorbing structure or tissue must get rid of that energy in some way. The manner in which this energy is dissipated causes the different biological effects on tissue that have been previously discussed.

The key physical event is absorption. Consistent, reproducible absorption in tissue is important to provide for a consistent outcome during medical therapy and surgical manipulation of tissues. Water is a major component of every soft tissue in the body, making up between 87% and 92% of the target pigment that CO_2 laser energy can be imparted to in the tissue. Since water so efficiently absorbs CO_2 lasers' light, most soft tissue is affected in an equal and reproducible way regardless of the type of delivery system. This makes for a very reliable and consistent tissue interaction for the clinician. It also allows for maximal expectation of reproducible clinical outcomes, especially between different clinicians using various CO_2 platforms.

Hemoglobin has a very high absorption rate in the violet and blue/green portions of the visible spectrum. The absorption starts to decline in the red region of the spectrum. This is why hemoglobin is red (it does not absorb red light but instead reflects it away from its surface). For this reason using an argon laser that emits blue/green light as the primary treatment for vascular lesions is ideal. Hemoglobin absorbs blue/green light and converts it into thermal energy, which contracts the blood vessel by denaturing its endothelial lining. This causes the local removal of the blood vessel. It is important to restate that fact. This wavelength region also has an increased possibility of beam scatter and transmission unless the laser is very precisely controlled and confined to the target tissue area during the treatment. Laser energy and its subsequent heating event will radiate in all directions and may destroy the overlying skin layers if not well controlled.

Some lasers, like the Neodymium-YAG (Nd:YAG) and the Diode (600 nm to 980 nm) have light energy that is very poorly absorbed by hemoglobin, water, and other body pigments. This type of laser energy relies on a multiple pigment effect to produce a general tissue interaction. Depending on the representative quantities of each pigment in a given tissue, a much greater variation in tissue interaction and reduced expected reproducible tissue events are more common. This is a key reason why the Nd:YAG and Diode laser light will penetrate and scatter much more deeply into tissue.

The selection of the correct laser for a particular clinical procedure requires an understanding of the absorptive as well as the reflective, scattering, and transmitting properties of the target tissue. It is therefore critical that the clinician has a clear understanding of the photobiologic, photochemical, and photothermal effects of the selected laser on the target pigment and thus the target tissue and surrounding tissues.

Chapter 4
Types of Laser-Tissue Interaction Related to the Rate of Heat Transfer Through Soft Tissue

"What power setting should I use for this procedure?" is the most common question a new laser surgeon may ask. The fact is, depending on the type of procedure and type of laser energy to be used, there is no one correct answer. The laser-tissue interaction concepts advanced herein are a guide to the surgical judgments that must be made to produce the desired effect in tissue. There is clearly a range of produced effects that depend on many factors: wavelength of energy used, power density applied, target tissue composition, elapsed time of exposure to radiation, and hand speed of the surgeon. There is as much art to successful surgery as there is science. The artistic aspects of veterinary soft tissue laser surgery are detailed in Chapter 8 and the Case Studies. Here we focus on the basic physical science of heat energy transfer through soft tissue and the resulting laser–tissue interactions.

Power Density

We feel that power density is the most important element of laser physics for the veterinary laser surgeon to comprehend. Understanding this concept fully will substantially increase the ability of the surgeon to achieve consistent, reproducible, and reliable therapeutic outcomes for the patient. As stated previously, laser-tissue interaction depends greatly on wavelength. The laser's effect depends on the power placed into the system to produce the photons and the power concentrated within the photons.

Power is usually expressed in watts on equipment settings. Any time laser energy is applied to tissue to produce a desired effect and time is also a factor, the term "joule" is used. A joule is defined as a watt-second; it is the amount of time power is applied to a target tissue to produce a cumulative effect. The aperture spot size, also known as the focal spot, results in the concentration of energy within an area producing a power density, expressed as watts/cm^2. The advantage of a small focal spot size with adequate power applied over a specific time is optimal vaporization of the target tissue. This also produces less secondary collateral thermal damage to tissue. Fewer cells are affected, damaged, or destroyed at the margins of an incision made using higher power density. When a deep laser trough is required, a small spot size is advantageous in that it concentrates a high amount of energy into the tissue due to extremely high amounts of excess fluence and rapid vaporization in that zone. When tissue heating or coagulation rather than vaporization is to be the effect, a larger spot size increases the area of the beam and thus reduces the total power density to the tissue. The energy is dispersed over a larger area, thus reducing fluence deposited to the target tissue. (Figure 4-1)

Figure 4-1 Note the contrast in the depicted zones of photothermolytic activity in these two laser beams, one with low power density and the other with high power density. The beam on the left has a lower power density and produces a shallower crater with wide zones of carbonization, thermal necrosis, and heat conduction. The beam on the right has a high power density and produces a deeper crater due to its greater penetration depth. This crater will have minimal tissue damage from thermal conduction and thin zones of carbonization and thermal necrosis. Lower power density is desirable for coagulation, and higher power density is desirable for ablation and incision.

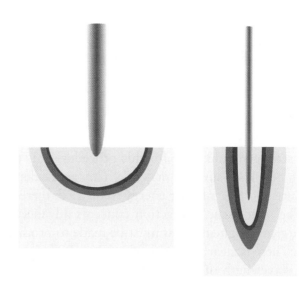

It is clear, then, that the power density can be affected by three main components under the clinician's control: power, time, and spot size. Knowing intuitively how these components interact will maximize the potential for a positive therapeutic outcome to the patient. The interplay of spot size, distance from focal area, angle of incidence, hand speed, power, and time are the critical variables all competent laser surgeons need to understand. As the spot size decreases while the power remains constant, the power density (power per unit area) must necessarily increase. Conversely, as spot size grows from small to large, either by changing aperture openings or altering the distance from the target tissue, the power density will diminish. The distance of the laser focusing tip or handpiece from the target tissue has an inverse relationship to the amount of energy imparted on the target tissue. Note that we are talking about a focused laser beam. This is because a focused beam has an optimal focal distance of maximal power density known as a focal area. Power density then decreases as the beam converges or diverges away from this area in either direction. Collimated beams that do not have focusing capabilities have a consistent or flat-line effect on power density to the target tissue. In this case, distance does not play a role in the power density transmitted to the tissue. (Figure 4-2)

What does this mean to the target tissues, clinically speaking? If the clinical objective is to make a rapid zone of vaporization, the laser surgeon should use a very small spot size with a high power density. This will provide adequate power density to produce vaporization and allow for rapid laser troughing deep into the tissues. It will also allow most of the heat generation to be removed in the plume and away from the surrounding tissue. If the intent is to ablate more superficially or to cause heating, denaturation, or coagulation of protein and collagen, then a larger spot size that produces a lower power density should be used. Be aware that an increase in char and the potential for peripheral thermal conduction occurs in this scenario. The clinician can therefore control the kind of effect produced in the target tissue by manipulating the distance, spot size, or power settings on the laser. It is very important to recognize this abil-

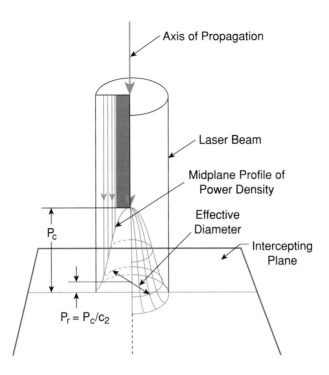

Axis of Propagation

Laser Beam

Midplane Profile of
Power Density

Effective
Diameter

Intercepting
Plane

P_c

$P_r = P_c/c_2$

Figure 4-2 A collimated laser beam travels unchanged along its path of propagation indefinitely until it strikes another object. Changing the distance from the point of origin to the intercepting plane does not change the power density of a collimated beam.

ity, so the clinician will be able to get the most out of the device and produce the best clinical results for the patient. Please note that in cases where fixed crystal fibers are being used, *e.g.*, Nd:YAG and diode lasers, the variation in power density is divided into power settings in the contact mode or non-contact mode of these devices. This is because the laser-to-tissue distance is zero in contact mode, eliminating distance as a variable. Therefore, only the level of power imparted on the system can be altered to increase or decrease the power density.

Laser radiation must be converted into another form of energy to produce therapeutic effects when it interacts with the target tissue. Laser-tissue interactions are categorized according to whether laser energy is converted into heat (photothermal), chemical energy (photochemical), or acoustic mechanical effect (photodisruptive) energy. In the tissue, these events are not mutually exclusive and may affect tissue in concert or independently.

Photothermolysis is the basic mechanism of laser-tissue interaction. That is, the radiant energy delivered by a laser beam is absorbed by its target and transformed into heat energy that causes a rise in the tissue's temperature. There are power density thresholds that must be reached before effects of rising temperature take place in the tissue. Since other effects may occur at higher and higher thresholds, the surgeon must apply the appropriate power density to achieve the desired threshold without exceeding the threshold for the next higher, undesired level. If a surgeon needs to coagulate tissue, then the power density of the beam must be high enough to exceed the threshold for irreversible thermal damage, but not so high as to cause vaporization. Likewise, a surgeon who is vaporizing tissue must avoid both char formation and coagulation. In this case, a power density should be selected that exceeds both the thresholds of coagulation and vaporization but not the threshold of carbonization. These thresholds depend strongly on wavelength, power density, and tissue composition. This subject is covered in great detail in Chapter 2.

For the purposes of simplicity and practicality, the CO_2 laser-tissue interaction will be used for the discussions in this chapter. The following are the basic guidelines for laser energy properties within soft tissue that any laser surgeon must understand. The 10,600 nm wavelength is strongly absorbed by water, which makes it an ideal laser for soft tissue surgical applications. As long as the laser surgeon has a complete working knowledge of the wavelength applied and expected results, consistent results should be attainable within the limits of any wavelength, but especially with CO_2 energy. The boiling point of water, 100°C, is reached rather quickly when power densities above 1,500 W/cm² (power density) are applied, and produces the transformation of liquid water to steam vapor. Above 1,500 W/cm², the laser will consistently cause boiling. Below 10 W/cm², only warming of the water will occur. Between 100 W/cm² and 1,500 W/cm², a mixture of warming and vaporization will occur. Within soft tissue, these thresholds are almost equivalent. Between 10 W/cm² and 1,500 W/cm², a mixture of photopyrolysis and photovaporolysis will occur. Below 10 W/cm², only warming of the tissues, or photopyrolysis, will occur. Above 1,500 W/cm², complete photovaporolysis occurs.

The mechanism of vaporization of soft tissue by a laser beam is the sudden boiling of histologic water to form steam. This intra-cellular steam expands rapidly and ruptures the relatively weak cell membranes that previously confined it. The solid residue of cells and connective tissue are dehydrated and ejected from the impact zone of the laser beam and may actually ignite or burn, forming a plume of smoke. The temperature of the area not vaporized will be ≤100°C, and falls away exponentially with distance. As long as the steam vapor can escape from the boiling surface of the tissue, the tissue near the vaporized area is minimally damaged by thermal conduction through it. Fourier's law of thermal conduction, as applied to soft tissue, can be used to calculate the rate of thermal power density removal, and is given by:

$$P_{th} = - c_t \, (dT/dz)$$

where c_t is the thermal conductivity of tissue {(6.92 x 10⁻³ W/cm⁻¹ °C⁻¹) x % hydration}, T is the temperature at the surface of the tissue, z is the depth below this surface, and dT/dz is the temperature gradient at the tissue surface. Calculations based on experiments with soft tissues give this rate as 10 W/cm² to 30 W/cm². Therefore, if the applied power density in the beam is far above the rate of thermal power density removal, the vaporized tissue can be quickly removed before the flow of heat to adjacent tissue can cause significant coagulation. The concept of tissue cooling and thermal relaxation will be discussed later.

The ideal surgical use of a precise, incisional CO_2 laser does not depend on power density above the vaporization threshold of 100 W/cm². A CO_2 laser properly produces incisions with little or no heating of surrounding tissues due to the rapid vaporization of the target tissue and minimal thermal conduction to surrounding tissue. Any heating of tissue requires a definite temperature transfer time. This temperature transfer time depends on physical properties such as the specific heat of the target tissue, its thermal conductivity, its coefficient of radiant energy absorption, and its mass density or water content.

The specific heat of water, h, is the radiant energy absorbed per unit volume of tissue. One fundamental physical fact about pure water is that it requires 253 J/cm^3 to raise the temperature from 37°C to 100°C. The latent heat of vaporization of pure water, h_v, is 2,163 J/cm^3, which is the heat required to vaporize one unit volume of water at 100°C from water to steam. The water content of tissues, a proportion referred to as w, is generally 70% to 90%. Recalling that fluence, f, is the radiant energy delivered to tissue over a unit area, we can also express fluence as the time-integral of power density during the time, T_p, of the laser pulse:

$$f = \int_0^{\tau_p} P_o \, dt \qquad \text{(Figure 4-3)}$$

Thus, the absorption coefficient, a, can be expressed as the ratio of the specific heat of water, h, over the fluence at a given wavelength:

$$a = h / f$$

The absorption coefficient of histologic water targeted by a CO_2 laser is 770 cm^{-1}. The role of the absorption coefficient, a, in laser-tissue interaction is fundamental to the appropriate choice of wavelength for a particular surgical use.

For the purposes of understanding how radiant energy is absorbed by tissue to causes a rise in temperature, we will assume that a hypothetical perfect pulse of constant power density is delivered to tissue containing 100% water. We will assume a CO_2 laser is used to produce the pulse of a Gaussian beam, TEM_{00}. We will also assume that the radiant pulse reaches peak power instantly, and that at the end of the pulse the radiant power is instantly quenched to zero. Under these hypothetical conditions, exaggerated for clarity, the fluence and absorption density both rise linearly with time from the start of the pulse. As the fluence increases, the

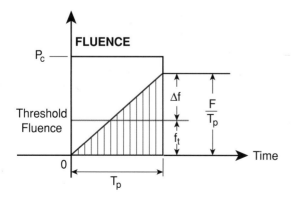

Figure 4-3 A graphical illustration of the time integral of power density, or fluence. Assuming a steady rate of energy deposition, the shaded area represents total fluence. Steeper curves are produced by higher power density, and curves with low slope may represent sub-ablation threshold power densities.

temperature of the tissue will increase proportionally to the absorption coefficient at that wavelength. The histologic water will boil at the instant when the threshold of fluence has been delivered. From the previous equation, this threshold fluence is the sum of:

$$f_t = (253 \text{ J/cm}^3) \,/\, a = 328 \text{ mJ/cm}^2$$

or the energy density required to raise the temperature of pure water from 37°C to 100°C plus

$$f_v = (2163 \text{ J/cm}^3) \,/\, a = 2809 \text{ mJ/cm}^2$$

or the energy density required to vaporize water at 100°C into steam, and is a total of 3,137 mJ/cm².

Note that the absorption density, *h*, and the absorption coefficient, *a*, are both dependent on the same concentration of histologic water and are adjusted proportionally to that constant, w. The threshold fluence, f_t, however, is independent of the concentration of water within tissue:

$$h_w = [w] \, h$$

$$a_w = [w] \, a$$

$$f_t = h_w \,/\, a_w$$

If sufficient fluence is delivered to exceed this threshold and vaporization occurs due to this excess fluence, Δf, then a kerf will be created at the tissue surface that has a 3-D Gaussian profile, much like a crater. This is often referred to as the zone of vaporization and is often designated as a laser trough (Figure 4-4). The diameter of this crater is referred to as the

Figure 4-4 A tissue kerf is produced by a Gaussian laser beam that moves in a given direction, x, in tissue. Its depth, z, is dependant on excess deposited fluence. Its width, y, is dependant on the effective diameter of the beam. The kerf length is a result of the time that the beam moves at velocity, v. Intuitively, slower speeds create greater penetration depth but deposit more fluence to a given area. Faster speeds will not allow excess fluence to be deposited at depth, and will require higher power density to achieve the ablation threshold. To avoid excess char formation, a surgeon with rapid handspeed may require high power to make incisions and a surgeon with slow handspeed should use lower power when creating incisions.

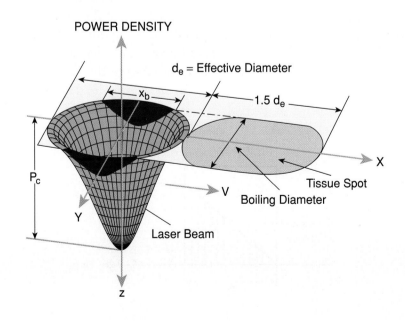

boiling diameter of the beam, and its depth at the center, z_c, is directly related to the excess fluence:

$$z_c = (f_v - f_t)/ h_v = \Delta f_c / h_v$$

As a reminder, the boiling diameter is generally produced where the power density greatly exceeds 100 W/cm².

At the instant vaporization occurs due to the excess fluence, a plume of desiccated material is ejected from the crater, taking much of the heat of vaporization with it. Transfer of heat outside the zone of vaporization occurs by thermal conduction through the tissue, and may be accentuated by sub-threshold fluence deposited at the tissue. It is axiomatic that tissues farther away from the boiling diameter will experience less temperature change compared to tissues closer to the boiling diameter. This change in temperature with distance from the crater can be calculated from Fourier's law of thermal conduction, or extrapolated from the graphical depiction of a curve based on distance vs. temperature. The initial slope of the curve of temperature vs. ablation depth, z_c, is such that the tangent to the curve intersects the z-axis at a depth 1/a, and the temperature axis at 100°C (Figure 4-5).

The cumulative effects of radiant energy on tissue are time-dependent. Ideally, as described previously, there is no conduction of heat to surrounding tissues. No heat is conducted through tissue in this case because all of the fluence is instantaneously above threshold. Any heat is abducted via ejected steam and desiccated cellular residue. In contrast, when sub-threshold fluence is delivered, the tissue only becomes warmed and does not vaporize. Some of this heat may be high enough to cause coagulation; this occurs within the zone of thermal necrosis. There is the potential for regeneration and viability at all points distant from the center of the beam where the tissue is warmed but not excessively. This is the zone of thermal conduction and repair. Repeated doses of sub-threshold fluence will cause greater areas of thermal necrosis and contribute greatly to undesirable surgical outcomes unless the goal is tissue coagulation. Repeated doses of supra-threshold fluence will create a greater depth of the zone of

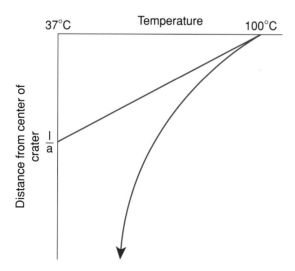

Figure 4-5 The change in temperature with distance from the center of a laser-induced vaporization crater can be extrapolated from this curve of temperature vs. distance. Note the initial slope of the curve is such that the tangent to it intersects the distance axis at a depth 1/a, and the temperature axis at 100°C.

vaporization and minimal thermal conduction, which is ideal for incisions and ablations but not for cauterization of larger vessels.

Photothermal Effect (Heat)

Photothermal effects occur when laser light is absorbed by tissue and converted into heat energy within the target tissue. This results in a rise in the target tissue temperature. As was discussed earlier, a variety of tissue effects can be seen, based on the temperature reached. CO_2 wavelengths in the far infrared range specifically affect the water component of the pigment of the target tissue. As the effected pigment, water plays a predominant role in the absorption of laser energy. It is heated directly with laser energy and at the correct power density, boils almost instantaneously on an intra-cellular level. This produces an explosive event to the target tissue and vaporization is achieved. Other molecules may then be indirectly heated via heat conduction from the point of the vaporization event. Other tissue components (hemoglobin, melanin, proteins, and others), as discussed before, may also absorb energy at specific infrared wavelengths. They can and do play an important role in the tissue heating process.

The absorption of laser energy in any tissue is the sum of the absorption of each of the tissue components coupled with the absorption coefficient of the amount of water in the tissue. A perfect example of this is the effective absorption of CO_2 laser light, which is heavily absorbed by water in soft tissue. Its extinction depth is approximately 0.030 mm. The extinction depth for the Nd:YAG laser light, which is less efficiently absorbed by water, is about 1 mm to 3 mm.

The control of target tissue heating and limitations to peripheral thermal tissue injury are of paramount importance for proper therapeutic outcomes when using laser energy. As the temperature in the target tissue rises to 37°C to 60°C, the tissue starts to retract and conformational changes occur. With a temperature between 60° and 90°C, there is protein denaturization and coagulation. From 90°C to 100°C, carbonization and tissue burning occurs. Above 100°C, the tissue is vaporized and ablated. Ideally, from a clinical point of view, the clinician should be able to stop the heating process at any one of these thermal ranges to produce the desired clinical result. Understanding the factors that control target-tissue-to-laser effects is key to placing this knowledge into action. Experienced laser clinicians can visually determine the effect of the specific laser energy on the target tissue. This allows the clinician to stop the heating at the desired point. It is therefore equally important for clinicians who plan to use lasers to complete some hands-on course work so they better understand the visual considerations. It is also important to understand how to maximize the vaporization and ablative effects of laser energy while minimizing heating and denaturing events and vice versa.

Laser surgeons must also remember that heat radiates outward in all directions from the target area. Around the laser trough (the depression left after tissue is vaporized from a specific area) produced by tissue vaporization, there will be zones of carbonization, vacuolization, and edema as the heat is dissipated. The tissue in the zones of vacuolization and edema may be irreversibly affected and eventually necrose and slough out. This is especially true if poor technique, inappropriate energy, or incorrect laser selection is implemented. The host tissue may repair the area of affected tissue. This is only possible if minimal peripheral tissue injury is produced and the thermal relaxation time of the target tissue is satisfied. The clinician's ability to optimally vaporize the tissue will maximize the removal of heat in the plume. This effectively limits or eliminates peripheral heat transfer to the surrounding tissue. Clinicians who do not clearly understand laser energy will not necessarily produce a nice clean laser trough by vaporization, and may leave peripheral tissue completely or minimally unaffected.

The objective of laser therapy must be to minimize as much as possible the secondary zones of thermal necrosis and injury, while maximizing tissue removal in the form of vaporization. For this reason it is important to again review the factors that interact with and direct laser energy to provide a superior tissue interactive outcome.

Thermal Relaxation Time

One of the most important concepts to grasp for appropriate application of laser energy is the tissue *thermal relaxation time*. Thermal relaxation time is the time necessary for target tissue to cool down by 50% through transfer of heat to surrounding tissues via thermal diffusion or other heat dissipation events discussed below. Optimally, the thermal relaxation time is instantaneous, leaving no peripheral thermal effect on the non-targeted tissue. Very short thermal relaxation times are typically identified when CO_2 laser energy is used at an appropriate distance, spot size, energy level, and energy release from the laser handpiece. This type of laser energy has the greatest application to most soft tissue procedures because of its consistent and reproducible effect. Thermal relaxation optimization is critical to avoiding secondary peripheral tissue effects. The clinician must understand the physical effect of the wavelength of laser energy being used on the target tissue and surrounding tissue structures. This will help avoid unwanted peripheral tissue interactions and unfavorable surgical and therapeutic outcomes.

To a much lesser extent, in most cases the removal or transfer of heat can be affected by a number of other energy transferring events: photochemistry, fluorescence, photoablation, ionization, and to an even more miniscule extent, plasma formation and biostimulation, which play secondary roles in laser energy transfer or release.

When ablating tissue with a laser, surrounding tissues will experience a change in temperature that occurs during a specified period of time. This adjacent zone of thermal damage can be minimized by reducing the time that tissues are exposed to a laser beam. This can be achieved by using a high power density applied to the target in a series of very short pulses with longer periods of rest (no energy input), allowing tissue to cool in between pulses. Pulsing a laser in this manner is an effective way to minimize thermal injury to tissues adjacent to the vaporized target. Remember that pulsing laser energy will, by itself, be only one adjunct factor in a whole series of steps to minimize peripheral thermal injury. Most commercially available CO_2 lasers have at least one pulse mode setting. Pulse mode settings are quantified by milliseconds; 1,000 msec = 1 second.

When the pulse of energy delivered from the laser beam has ended, the tissue will dissipate any heat, or cool off, by thermal conduction to surrounding tissue. How long does this take? It is useful to calculate the thermal relaxation time of the volume of tissue that was irradiated. Thermal relaxation time depends on the heated volume of tissue and its thermal conductivity. It is defined as the time required for a unit volume of tissue to cool down to one half of its maximum temperature during the irradiation, and can be calculated from:

$$1 / t_r = 4 \, \delta \, a^2$$

where t_r is the calculated thermal relaxation time, *a* is the absorption coefficient of tissue at that wavelength, and δ is a parameter named the *thermal diffusivity* of tissue, equal to 1.3×10^{-3} cm^2/s. For a CO_2 laser used on typical soft tissue, the thermal relaxation time can be calculated to be approximately 325 µs.

It follows then, that if the duration of a laser pulse to tissue is made shorter than the thermal relaxation time, a rise in temperature of non-irradiated surrounding tissue can be precluded or held below the threshold of fluence for thermal necrosis. Likewise, maximum vaporization with minimal thermal conduction can be achieved if several successive pulses are delivered to tissue and are restricted to a pulse time shorter than t_r and have an interval of time between pulses much greater than t_r. This desirable process is called *superpulsing*, and it is characterized by repetitive laser energy delivery and rest periods measured in microseconds.

Mechanically Altered Laser-Tissue Interaction

Laser surgeons must understand the mechanical alterations to laser energy delivery to explore its potential therapeutic benefits. Mechanical and computer-assisted delivery of laser energy can provide more effective vaporization, tissue/energy transfer, and optimal target tissue effect, with minimal peripheral thermal effects. These mechanical and computer-assisted effects are: continuous wave (CW), pulse wave (PW), and superpulse wave (SP).

Continuous Wave

When a laser, for example a CO_2 laser, is operating in the continuous wave mode (CW), laser energy is continually released through an open shutter during activation. The faceplate power setting relates the actual power release of the device in real time.

Pulsed Wave

The pulsed wave mode (PW) allows laser energy to be released in repeated bursts of duration specified by computer manipulation of the shutter. The peak pulses of the laser emission in this mode are substantially higher than the average power release over time. There are short periods during the lasing process in which no beam is released. This repeated pulse duration is measured in milliseconds, with the pulsed rate provided in pulses per second or Hz. This mode allows higher peak power into the target tissue. The added benefit is cooling of the peripheral tissue between pulses, which maximizes vaporization effects and minimizes thermal accumulation, which reduces heat trauma over time.

Superpulse Wave

The superpulse mode (SP) provides bursts of laser energy at even higher peaks (see Figure 1–18). This is accompanied by shorter pulse duration in the microsecond range. Equivalent pauses in the energy release are also supplied via computer-controlled release of the laser beam. The energy release pulses are well within the thermal relaxation time of the peripheral tissue. This higher peak energy release, coupled with increased rate of pulse repetition, effectively eliminates heat accumulation in the peripheral tissue.

Superpulse waveforms minimize thermal damage to normal tissue adjacent to CO_2 laser surgical sites. Ideally, this mode delivers extremely high fluence at an extremely rapid rate, thus instantaneously vaporizing tissue without allowing time for thermal conduction through the tissue. The entire pulse sequence, from initiation to termination, must occur in less time than the thermal relaxation time of the tissue for that wavelength. The peak power that is produced in superpulse mode is much greater than the average power the laser is capable of producing in continuous mode delivery. This peak power delivery is followed by a rapidly declining curve of power with respect to time. Because it is impossible for a mechanical shutter to support this speed of energy pulsing, an alternate approach was invented.

AC-excited Superpulse Waveform

A CO_2 laser resonant cavity is filled with a proprietary mixture of CO_2, N_2, and He gas. Alternating electrical current can be efficiently managed by solid state switching devises run by computer software to create pumped pulses of excitation energy in the laser medium, releasing finite packages of photons. Rapid peak total increases in electrical energy are followed by an equal period of zero excitation energy. This creates the pumping pattern that allows superpulsing to occur from the laser resonant cavity. At the instant the cavity receives strong pumping, the laser produces high power density radiation for the duration of the pulse, T_p. When the RF electrical output is suddenly zero, the laser also immediately discontinues power output as well, T_o, although there is a definite short period of time during which fluence rapidly diminishes toward zero (T_p to T_o). The superpulse waveform of power density with respect to time appears rectangular in its output form, with a slightly decreasing angle to its peak power output level. The laser produces a distinctive superpulse "buzz" as these unique energy packets are released. When using a CO_2

laser in homogenous soft tissue, the thermal relaxation time is calculated to be 325 μs. To satisfy the criteria for a superpulse waveform, a single isolated superpulse wave must be generated in less than that period of time to fall within the thermal relaxation time of the tissue. Peak energy output is generally over 200 mJ and lasts less than 325 μs to achieve these tissue/laser effects.

Some lasers are equipped with *ultrapulse* mode of delivery, which requires RF electrical current excitation of the medium. These lasers typically produce a *minimum* of 500 mJ within 50 μs, and maintain fluence at that level until the pumping ceases. The ultrapulse waveform of power density vs. time also appears rectangular, with a slightly decreasing angle to its peak power output level. The total amount of energy that an ultrapulsing laser delivers is significantly greater than that of an RF-excited superpulsing laser. There is an even greater excess of fluence above threshold that an ultrapulsed laser delivers to tissue during vaporization. This means that there is even less thermal necrosis to adjacent tissues caused by an ultrapulsed CO_2 laser, compared to any superpulsed laser (Figure 4-6).

DC-excited Superpulse Waveform

Older CO_2 lasers that produced a superpulse pattern used DC electricity to excite the medium. Devices in these lasers caused rapid cyclical on-and-off switching of current. The resulting superpulse waveform of power density vs. time is multi-exponential when excited by switched DC current. Notice that during DC pumping the power output reaches peak before the conclusion of the excitation period, T_p, at about 100 μs. The power then declines exponentially until the end of the pump duration. Furthermore, power output continues for a short period of time following pumping and also declines exponentially toward zero at a slower rate. This area has been referred to as a *power output tail* and is characteristic of the DC-excited superpulse waveform.

A sudden strong pumping of the resonant cavity causes the first sharp

Figure 4-6 A comparison of power output vs. time of pulse delivery for both superpulse and ultrapulse waveforms. The ultrapulse waveform is characterized by delivery of power above the ablation threshold for about 90% of its pulse duration. The superpulse waveform is not as efficient. Note, however, that the duration of the superpulse waveform is within the thermal relaxation time of tissue. Either of these patterns enables superior incisive power, but the cost of ultrapulse lasers may be too high for most practitioners.

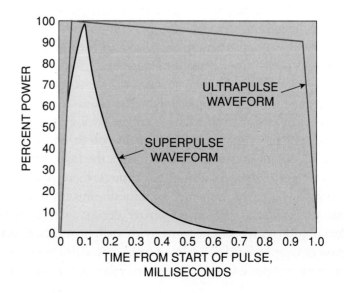

peak of laser energy to be produced. Within a few microseconds, the contents of the resonant cavity that were in the singlet laser level are found to be in the ground laser level state. This is a reflection of a profound population inversion that is rapidly reduced after the laser first produces a beam. The waveform abruptly loses power as the majority of molecules settle down to the ground state. Then, as the pumping suddenly stops, brief continued electrical discharge and the depletion of excited molecules causes exponentially reduced radiant output until it is zero. This process is repeated over and again several times per second to produce the superpulse waveform from a switched DC electrical current. It is more difficult to describe the important periods of time that characterize this waveform.

$f_s = 1/T_s$ = frequency of superpulses

T_p = time that driving voltage is applied during pumping pulse

Note that we can arbitrarily define the radiant output period, T_p, as the ratio of the total energy of the pulse over the peak power of the pulse in the DC-excited superpulse waveform of power density vs. time. The frequency of repetition of the pulses, f_r, is the same. At the end of T_p, fluence continues to be deposited to the tissues. This energy is generally sub-threshold for vaporization and instead causes the temperature of the target tissues to rise. If a long enough period of time elapses between pulses, the tissues can cool to a greater degree and thus experience less thermal injury. However, if the frequency of the train of superpulses increases, there will be less time for tissue cooling between superpulses and more thermal necrosis will occur due to the accumulation of thermal energy within the surrounding tissues. The ratio of the output time, T_p, over the repetition period of the superpulse, T_s, is known as the *duty factor*; duty factor = T_p / T_r

Duty Factor

Comparing duty factors demonstrates the need to keep this parameter low. We will examine four superpulsed lasers at duty factors of 5%, 10%, 20%, and 40% (Figure 4-7). Assume that the temperature at a point near the vaporization crater will increase as a result of tissue vaporization. This heat depends on both sub-threshold fluence at that point and thermal conduction through the tissue. It is clear that at a duty factor of 40% there is a progressive increase in temperature and an accumulation of heat that results from the inability of the tissue to cool between superpulses. This increase in temperature is lower when a duty factor of 20% is used and lower still with a duty factor of 10%. When a theoretical duty factor of 5% is used, or $T_p / T_r = 1 / 20$, it is clear that there should be no accumulation of heat surrounding the laser trough. Prior to the next superpulse of energy output, the tissue has already cooled down to its original temperature. Thus, thermal necrosis is obviated and a better surgical outcome consistent with scalpel blade characteristics (considered the gold standard for incisions) is expected from the incision. Ideally, a superpulsed laser should have a duty factor less than 5%, but this just is not so. Many commercial lasers may have duty factors of 25% or more!

The principal concept is that superpulsing provides less accumulation of heat to surrounding tissues compared to continuous laser delivery, but not zero. So it is important to note that the gold standard for incisional effect, the scalpel blade, can be approximated, but not fully realized with current lasers. Newer diamond scalpel blades delivering CO_2 or diode laser energy may provide the realization and tactile feel some clinicians strive for with current lasers. The tradeoff is the improvement in hemostasis, reduction in swelling, and reduction in nociceptor stimulation at the surgical site that appropriate laser energy can provide.

Superpulsing is not the same as intermittently repeating a continuous laser. Most lasers have the ability to deliver power in an interrupted fashion, known as pulsing or wave chopping. The frequency of these pulses ranges from 2 Hz to 200 Hz. Note that the period of time that a pulsed laser delivers energy is at least 5 msec per pulse, which is at least ten times the thermal relaxation time of tissue. This means that a great deal of heat is deposited in the target tissue for the period of time the tissue is exposed to laser energy. This then results in the creation of char due to the combustion of desiccated tissue residues. As previously described, char absorbs all wavelengths of laser energy very efficiently. The excess energy absorbed by the char is transformed to heat, which further increases the temperature of the surrounding tissues. If unchecked (via mechanical removal of the accumulated char), it is more likely that continued thermal

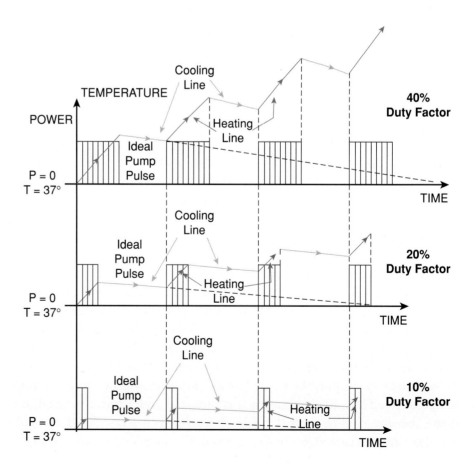

Figure 4-7 A comparison of the accumulation of heat within tissue in response to laser vaporization using three different duty factors. Note the general trend of increasing temperature with higher duty factors. A duty factor of 5% or less produces negligible accumulation of heat and is not depicted in this figure.

injury will occur with each pass of the laser energy over the char. Minimizing the pulse time, maximizing the power, and optimizing the period of time between continuous pulses will diminish these cumulative effects. Again, superpulsing is more appropriate for incising tissues because the time of the vaporizing pulse is less than the thermal relaxation time of tissue.

The key feature of superpulse mode is the rapid generation of high power density that can be used for photovaporolysis without conduction of heat to surrounding tissues. This occurs because the time period of the pulse, T_p, is engineered to be less than the thermal relaxation time. The heat conduction to surrounding tissue is minimized because the tissue absorbs all radiant energy during the pulse, and there is no time during which sub-threshold fluence is deposited to cause any significant thermal conduction to occur. Vaporizing parameters may be achieved by suitably prolonging the period of time between superpulses near ideal tissue. A CO_2 laser with a superpulse mode and a small duty factor is an ideal tissue-cutting tool, but a poor coagulation tool.

Photonic energy can also be absorbed and altered by other properties. These must be considered when using lasers to do therapeutic work on tissue. While these collective effects may be minimal at vaporization thresholds, other photonic tissue effects can themselves bear great importance for future diagnostic and therapeutic protocols and equipment.

Photochemistry

Photon energy may also be absorbed and thus dissipated by photochemistry effects on the target tissue. The basic concept of photochemistry is that certain molecules, both natural and applied, that reside in the target tissue can function as photosensitizers effecting energy uptake by the target tissue. The presence of these photosensitizers in certain cells causes them to be increasingly vulnerable to light of an appropriate wavelength and intensity. The action of these photosensitizers allows absorption of photons more specifically by these tissues than surrounding tissues. The excited photosensitizer subsequently reacts with other molecular substrates in the target tissue, in most cases oxygen, to produce singlet free radical oxygen units, which cause irreversible free radical oxidation on some of the essential cellular components. In most cases all of this occurs without significant generation of heat in the target tissue. This has given rise to photodynamic therapies that use specific photosensitizers react to specific laser energy wavelengths. Visible light lasers make up the bulk of this wavelength for use in photosensitization therapy.

The most specific example of this mechanism has been in the treatment of cancer cells that have been tagged or sensitized with a photosensitizer such as a hematoporphyrin derivative. The mechanism of hematoporphyrin derivatives' preference to locate in malignant cells is still not fully understood but is likely related to specific protein receptor sites on the surface of cancer cells that have a higher affinity for uptake of the sensitizer. This can explain why the total time that hematoporphyrin derivatives are retained in malignant tissue is much longer than in nonmalignant tissue surrounding them. The sensitizing agent generally clears from non-cancerous tissue in 72 hours but is retained for extended periods by specific neoplastic cells. As a result, there is a window of time to cause the selective photodegradation of malignant tissue without significant alteration to adjacent normal tissue. It is also important to note that because of the wait time for clearance of these types of compounds. The individual or animal being treated must also stay away from visible (white) light. This is because, as discussed before, white light is made up of many wavelengths of light. Some of these also may be specific for uptake by the sensitizing material.

Fluorescence

Photon energy may also be dissipated as the re-emission of light. If this happens within 10^{-6} seconds after absorption, it is called fluorescence. The fluorescent photon is emitted as the excited fluorescent-emitting atom in the target tissue returns to the ground state. Because excess energy is primarily dissipated as heat by collisions with other atoms in the excited state the energy of the fluorescent photon is altered from that of the absorbed photon. This event can be adapted to make diagnoses. It is now used to determine the extent of superficial skin tumors and to detect occult lung tumors. Tumors may also be able to be tagged with atoms that can fluoresce, allowing clinicians to see the extent of a mass to a more specific and complete degree than ever before. In addition, devices that detect these fluorescence photons are used for non-invasive cholesterol monitoring and detection of certain vitamins and other body chemicals.

The only limit of detection is the ability to detect light, but with the advent of image intensifiers now under development becoming sensitive enough, it would theoretically be possible to detect just a few photons of light emitted from a single malignant cell. Laser-stimulated fluorescence can also be used analytically to scan large populations of cells flowing through a laser beam in a device known as a cytofluorometer. These are now used in the most advanced hemocytometers available. They allow a substance or tissue to move through it while continually applying to the tissue a wavelength of laser energy specific to the tissue to create fluorescence. Photo-receptive cells in the housing can pick up fluorescent photons emitted and identify the wavelength specific to the cell, tissue, or substance. This is being used to determine if malignant lymphocytes are present in blood and then selectively remove them.

Photoablation

The photoablative process consists of the direct breaking of intra-molecular bonds in polymeric chains caused by the absorption of high-energy ultraviolet photons. This is also known as photo-dissociation. The lasing materials of excimer lasers primarily produce this effect as they are excited dimers of unstable gases, usually a halogen and some rare element. The ultraviolet photons generated by these lasers possess so much energy that they will literally break apart molecular bonds before their energy can be dissipated as heat, thus reducing the tissue to its atomic constituents. Since ultraviolet radiation from 200 nm to 360 nm is well absorbed by most biological molecules with penetration depths of only a few microns, this feature is used to produce well defined, non-thermal cuts of very small width by excimer lasers currently used in corneal resurfacing procedures in human ophthalmology.

The treatment of a number of ocular disorders via the potential of changing the eye's refractive power by precisely removing corneal tissue without generating secondary heat effects is now well documented. Ablation of the corneal stroma with 193 nm of radiation has been shown to produce clean, non-thermal cuts. Thus, there is no peripheral heat to be transferred and no chance of destroying or damaging surrounding ocular tissue. This wavelength of energy also does not transmit or penetrate deeply so injury to other ocular structures such as the retina is eliminated. The advent of precise topical tissue mapping devices will allow even greater refinements in corneal resurfacing and stromal layer contouring. This laser may also have some applications in dermatology, neurosurgery, and orthopedics, where precise tissue removal without any thermal event would be highly desirable. The drawback is the very small amount of tissue that can be removed at one time with this process. As with the laser eye procedures, it takes thousands of laser firings in extremely rapid fashion under the control of a computer linked to a topographical corneal surface-mapping device to produce the desired effect.

Ionization

Ionization is the ejection of an electron from an atom. This is best understood in a thermonuclear energy release of ionizing radiation. It is generally felt that the individual photons generated from existing lasers do not have enough energy to cause the absorbing molecule to lose an electron. Investigation into X-ray lasers and free electron beam lasers (currently under development by the military) has developed the photon energy that would be sufficient, of course, to cause the ejection of an electron from a target molecule. While military applications are likely from this type of laser energy, there is currently limited therapeutic value in this form of energy transfer. If specific energy patterns can be produced that have selective interaction with only certain types of cells, such as cancer cells, then a new way of selectively destroying only atypical neoplastic cells may be possible.

Cavitation and Vacuolization

The energy generated by a Holmium laser at the point of energy/tissue convergence can produce a physical effect that is not associated with vaporization, but more likely cavitation and vacuolization due to a plasma wave formation. When these lasers are precisely focused on a small spot of tissue it is possible to generate a "plasma." Plasma is a gaseous-like cloud rich in free electrons. An intense acoustical shockwave is generated in the medium preceding the event location due to the sudden production

Chapter 5
Laser Systems, Wavelengths, and Technology Selection

Until recently in veterinary medicine, the laser was considered a device that held great potential but was in search of an application. Most medical lasers were extremely cumbersome, expensive, and difficult to maintain until 1996, when technology allowed smaller units to be manufactured. They were designed for human therapeutics, not the veterinary patient. However, the desire for minimally invasive surgical approaches, including incisions and laproscopic, intestinal endoscopic, perivisceral endoscopic, thoracoscopic, and intra-articular procedures, have sparked the use of laser energy by the veterinary community. This renewed interest is driving modifications in laser technology so it is better suited for the veterinary profession. Because universities and private research have lagged behind, general and specialty practitioners are currently driving the learning curve for the profession.. The number of procedures currently documented by the practicing veterinary community far exceeds university documentation of laser/tissue interaction. More veterinary universities are now obtaining lasers and beginning to use them in research clinics. This most likely will confirm the anecdotal results being obtained by thousands of practicing veterinarians.

Lasing medium is one of two terms in which biomedical lasers are described; the other is wavelength. The lasing medium may be gas, liquid, solid crystal, or diode. The following are examples of each type:

- Gas lasers: CO_2 with a wavelength of 10,600 nm
- Liquid lasers: Typically rhodamine dye, and tunable from 100 nm to 1,000 nm
- Solid crystal lasers: Neodymium:Yttridium-Aluminum-Garnet laser at 1,064 nm (Nd:YAG, 1,064 nm)
- Diode laser: Does not produce its light in a lasing chamber, but emits light when an electrical current is Passed through a solid-state chip. These diode lasers are available in various wavelengths ranging from 590 nm to 980 nm or higher wavelengths.

Many types of biomedical lasers are used in veterinary medicine today. Lasing medium, wavelength, and frequency determine each laser's absorption ability in differing biological tissues.

- CO_2 (10,600 nm) and Ho:YAG (2,100 nm)lasers: These are highly absorbed by water, making them perfect for tissue cutting, vaporization, and acoustical destruction. Because of high absorption by water, thermal injury to surrounding tissue is very superficial.

  CO_2 lasers have lateral thermal injury of 0.05 mm to 0.1 mm, and Ho:YAG lasers have lateral thermal injury of 0.1 mm to 1 mm. Because there is such minimal lateral thermal damage, injury to surrounding tissues is limited to what you see during application of the laser energy. Early CO_2 lasers were limited to delivery by cumbersome articulated arms, mirrors, and straight hollow wave-guide tubes. This significantly limited their practical application. Today, technology has given us the ability to send CO_2 laser light through highly reflective flexible wave-guides, leading to unlimited possibilities within the surgical arena. In the near future, development of halide optical fibers and smaller hollow wave-guides may make the CO_2 lasers applicable to endoscopic use as well.

The Ho:YAG laser can be delivered through flexible optical fibers, making it very useful for endoscopic procedures. The Ho:YAG laser is a pulsed laser, which creates much acoustical energy and makes it most suitable for lithotripsy.

- Solid-state diode lasers and Nd:YAG laser: The solid-state diode lasers in the 805 nm, 820 nm, and 970 nm range and the Nd:YAG laser at 1,064 nm are invisible wavelengths in the near infrared spectrum. These smaller, compact units emit wavelengths that are easily transmitted through small flexible optical fibers, allowing them to be used with most flexible and rigid endoscopes. The small flexible transmission fibers are made from glass silica or quartz. Vaporization of tissue can be accomplished in a non-contact mode. These transmission fibers, when trimmed or terminated in specialized tips, are used in a contact mode to accomplish cutting as well as tissue vaporization.

  The energy produced by diode lasers is not as easily absorbed by water as that produced by the CO_2 laser. This can result in a greater depth of thermal injury, especially if used in the non-contact mode. Minimal thermal damage occurs when the laser is used in the contact mode, rather than the non-contact mode. The shorter wavelength is better absorbed in hemoglobin, allowing efficient cutting and ablation of vascular tissues. The diode laser has better hemostasis of larger vessels than the CO_2 laser, also due to the better absorption by hemoglobin.

- Argon laser at 524 nm, KTP, and frequency-doubled Nd:YAG at 532 nm: These lasers emit visible green light highly absorbed by hemoglobin. Despite the absorption of light by hemoglobin, these wavelengths will readily pass through water, gastric fluid, aqueous or vitreous humor, and urine. These lasers are used both in contact and non-contact modes to precisely cut, vaporize, and coagulate tissues that are well perfused with blood. However, laser energy is severely attenuated if working in a bloody surgical field.

- Dye and diode lasers: These lasers, in the visible red spectrum wavelength of 635 nm to 675 nm, are used for photodynamic therapy. The patient is injected with a photosensitizer that is absorbed and concentrated in tumor cells, thus localizing the photodynamic effect. When the tumor is irradiated with laser light of the appropriate wavelength, a photochemical reaction generates reactive oxygen free radicals that kill the targeted tumor cells without seriously injuring the surrounding normal tissue. However, the extent of chemical-stimulated damage to the affected tissues often is not seen until 24 to 48 hours after treatment.

A number of wavelengths of laser energy currently are receiving consideration for use in the veterinary medical and surgical fields. The following is a list of those lasers and their respective wavelengths. The specific parameters of each of those lasers are also outlined.

Laser Delivery Systems

The following are a few comments and guidelines that can be considered or followed when selecting a laser technology to use or purchase. We have focused our practical use of lasers on the CO_2 and, to a lesser extent, diode wavelengths. A number of other wavelengths are being used at selected universities and in human surgical and dental fields. The reader should further investigate other laser wavelength applications only after gaining a complete knowledge of that wavelength's physical and tissue interactive properties through outside reading.

Table 5-1 Basic physical properties of current surgical lasers

Laser Type	Wavelength	Active Medium	Excitation	Power	Operating Mode	Target
Argon Ion Laser	488 nm, 514 nm	Ar^+ Gas	DC electrical discharge	<1 to >30 W	CW, PW	Hemoglobin
Krypton Ion Laser	476 nm, 521 nm, 568 nm, 647 nm	Kr^+ Gas				
Ruby Laser	694 nm (Red)	$Al_2O_3:Cr^{3+}$	Flash-lamp	Up to 10^9 W	Obligate pulsed (10 ps - ms)	Melanin
Alexandrite Laser	710 nm, 755 nm 820 nm	$BeAl_2O_4:Cr^{3+}$	Flash-lamp	Up to 100 W	CW, PW (100 ps - ms)	Melanin, hemoglobin
Dye Laser	308 - 1,300 nm	Liquid dye (Rhodamine 6G)	Flash-lamp/ Laser	Up to 10^6 W	Obligate pulsed	Photosensitizer, ureteral calculi
Semiconductor Diode Laser	590 - 5300 nm	Semiconductor (e.g. GaAlAs)	DC/AC	<1 to >30 W	CW, PW (ps - ms)	Hemoglobin, melanin, (water)
Nd:YAG Laser KTP Laser (frequency doubled Nd:YAG)	1,064 nm (KTP=532 nm)	Nd^{3+} in $Y_3Al_5O_{12}$	Krypton arc lamp	<1 to >100 W	CW, PW (20 ps - 5 ms)	Hemoglobin, melanin, (water)
Ho:YAG Laser	2,100 nm	Ho^{803+} in $Y_3Al_5O_{12}$	Xenon flash-lamp	Up to 10^4 W	Obligate pulsed	Water
Er:YAG Laser	2,936 nm	Er^{3+} in $Y_3Al_5O_{12}$	Xenon flash-lamp	Up to 10^5 W	Obligate pulsed	Water
CO_2 Laser	10,600 nm	Mixture of CO_2, N_2, He	DC/AC	<1 to >100 W	CW, PW, Superpulse (5 ms - 1 s)	Water
Excimer Laser		Dimer: Short-lived, excited ionized halogen/noble gas	High power AC			
ArF	193 nm			50 W	Obligate pulsed	Cornea, bone
KrCl	222 nm			50 W		
KrF	248 nm			100 W		
XeCl	308 nm			150 W		
XeF	351 nm			30 W		

Types of Medical Lasers

Many different types of biomedical lasers are in use today. Each instrument is usually acquired for a specific purpose, such as an incisional tool; excisional device; ablative device; photodisruption applications; or dermatological, endoscopic, otoscopic, or bronchoscopic applications. Overall, the use of laser energy can be an extremely precise method for tissue removal and a variety of laser wavelengths are in use today to a greater of lesser extent. The CO_2, diode, neodymium yttrium aluminum garnet (Nd:YAG), argon, KTP, ruby, and holmium wavelength lasers are some of the types used in veterinary and human medicine. The CO_2, diode and Nd:YAG lasers perform the majority of clinical practice duties, with the CO_2 holding the lion's share of current clinical applications.

Enhancements in laser application, wavelength specification, and delivery system are being made regularly, since they are closely aligned with advances in today's technology. Continuing upgrades to software and hardware applications also are advancing laser energy application. The ultimate goal for any laser user is to improve the final surgical or medical outcome for their patient's specific case. Having a working knowledge of the variety of laser wavelengths and their potentials can give the general practitioner an added appreciation for thinking outside the box with respect to available therapeutic and surgical case management. The following review of some of the currently used wavelengths of laser energy is provided to stimulate the reader to expand his or her view of currently accepted case management.

Carbon Dioxide Laser (10,600 nm)

The carbon dioxide laser wavelength is ideal for cutting and vaporization because, as previously stated, it is highly absorbed by water at the peak of the 6 μm absorption band. It can cut tissue cleanly when the beam is focused and can debulk tissue, providing adequate hemostasis when the beam is defocused. At the tissue interface, blood vessels less than 0.6 mm in diameter can be coagulated and sealed, which provides for improved surgical field visibility. Lymphatics are also sealed so postoperative edema may be reduced and secondary chemotactic factors initiating inflammatory responses are reduced.

Subjectively, there seems to be less pain associated with a laser incision and dissection. This observation could be due to the fact that smaller primary nociceptors are sealed and secondary nociceptors are not stimulated. The advent of superpulsed systems that typically can produce multiple packets of pulses—each one hundred microseconds in length—are able to provide significant energy to the tissue within that tissue's thermal relaxation time.

In addition, mechanical scanners can be adapted to the CO_2 to allow for large areas of tissue vaporization or ablation. This can be very advantageous for diffuse dermal masses, debridement, or granulation bed ablation. "What you see is what you get" when using carbon dioxide lasers. They are generally reported to have a very short learning curve, in the neighborhood of two to four weeks. As mentioned, energy delivery with a carbon dioxide laser can be provided through an articulated-arm with a series of mirrors for focusing the laser beam, or other delivery modalities, including hollow wave guides and compatible low OH optical fibers. These can offer energy delivery advantages in most clinical settings where access to the surgical field is limited.

Semiconductor Diode Lasers (810 nm to 980nm)

Recent engineering and commercial applications have allowed development of diode lasers with wavelengths varying from approximately 635 nm to 980 nm. Diode lasers used in veterinary medicine typically are in the 810 nm to 980 nm range. Newer technologies also allow diode lasers capable of emitting wavelengths in the mid-infrared range (2.1 *um*). Dual wavelength or dial-in diode lasers will become available in the near future.

The compact size and high efficiency of diode lasers offer the potential for economic advantages. Their relative small size is advantageous in facilities with limited space. Higher power diode lasers in the 25 watt to 50 watt range are available, and can provide significant cutting and coagulation ability in contact mode. These lasers currently provide up to 50 watts at approximately 810 nm, a wavelength that penetrates deeply into most types of soft tissue and provides superior hemostatic abilities to the CO_2 laser. It must be noted that increased peripheral tissue heating is a side effect in most cases. The lasers can be used with a variety of delivery fiber tips through an endoscope, otoscope, or bronchoscope. They can be used in non-contact mode for nonfocused deep tissue coagulation and vascular effect. Carbonization of the cleaved tip allows precise cutting or vaporization in a tissue contact mode.

Surgical diode lasers offer considerable advantages compared to Nd:YAG lasers with respect to reduced peripheral tissue interaction. They have a shallower depth of penetration (although still much larger then a CO_2 laser). They are smaller, lighter, and require less maintenance. They are considered extremely user-friendly once the learning curve (six to twelve weeks, due to increased variable tissue energy uptake factors) is completed, and can be more economical. This region of the near-infrared wavelength absorbs into the target tissue via several pigments in the target tissue. Diode lasers are absorbed by hemoglobin, melanin, oxyhemoglobin, and, to a lesser degree, water.

When using a near-infrared laser there are more variables related to laser-tissue interaction, especially more undesired peripheral thermal events. The zone of thermal necrosis can reach as high as 9 mm when the tissues are inadequately cooled. Tissue sloughing has been noted in some situations where an inexperienced user has applied excessive fluence. These lasers are sometimes referred to as WYDSCHY, or "What you don't see can hurt you." We consider the diode wavelength as an important next laser to add, once proficiency in using the CO_2 laser wavelength has been established. The diode laser can significantly complement CO_2 laser use in veterinary practice.

Nd:YAG Lasers (Neodymium Yttrium Aluminum Garnet; 1,064 nm)

The Nd:YAG or "YAG" laser differs greatly from the CO_2 laser because the wavelength transmits though tissue, in addition to the observed surface tissue effect. Nd:YAG lasers can deliver high powers of up to 100 watts through silicon-based optical transmitting fibers that can easily be inserted into working channels of standard GI endoscopes, fiberoptic otoscopes, and bronchoscopes. Power source requirements are also much greater, requiring a dedicated 220 AC line. Since the Nd:YAG laser has less specific absorption by water and hemoglobin than the carbon dioxide and argon lasers, the depth of thermal injury can exceed 3 mm in most tissues, which can be useful for coagulation of large volumes of tissue but also very dangerous to the untrained user. Fairly rapid tissue vaporization in non-contact mode is possible with a bare fiber, but collateral thermal injury may be substantial and produce unrewarding post-operative effects. Continuous wave or CW Nd:YAG lasers can be used with a contact mode with surgical precision to provide incision and coagulation. In this mode, little collateral thermal injury and good hemostasis can be achieved. Use of contact tips for endoscopic application is widely accepted, but some tips are too large to insert through flexible endoscopes. We feel that this laser wavelength should only be used by very knowledgeable, experienced laser practitioners, or in advanced university settings.

Frequency-Doubled-YAG Lasers ("KTP" or Potassium Titanyl Phosphate; 532 nm)

Frequency-doubled Nd:YAG lasers emit a visible green light and are basically equivalent to the argon lasers in many surgical and dermatological applications. There is little or no absorption by water at the 532 nm wavelength light. This gives an advantage when vascular tissue with ill-defined borders requires resection or ablation. This type of laser is not a very precise energy provider. Induced photothermolysis of tissue selectively stained with an indocyanine green chromatophore has also shown promise for selective coagulation and vaporization of tumors and contaminated wounds in recessed or surgically sensitive areas.

Visible Light-Emitting Lasers

There are currently no lasers in the visible light spectrum that are capable of effectively cutting tissue without significant thermal damage to the peripheral tissue zone. These types of lasers should not be considered for incisive work due to the delayed healing and scarring produced.

Argon Lasers (458 and 524 nm)

The blue-green light emitted from an argon laser is most significantly absorbed by hemoglobin, its primary tissue target. This makes it useful for specific removal of vascular lesions that are at a very shallow depth in the dermis (1 mm to 2 mm). Argon laser energy is not "seen" by most other tissues and thus transmits through water or other organic fluids. Bare fibers can be used in contact or non-contact modes for cutting, vaporization, or coagulation.

Ruby Lasers (694 nm)

This wavelength is primarily used as a device for removing tattoos and darkly pigmented birthmarks. There is currently limited value for this laser in general veterinary practice.

Holmium Lasers (2,100 nm)

Clinical holmium lasers are being used sparingly in veterinary medicine for arthroscopic surgery, lithotripsy, and very limited general surgery. Additional applications have been implemented for laser diskectomy by Dr. Ken Bartels at Oklahoma State University in a research setting. While this wavelength of laser interacts with water much like the CO_2 laser, it has a very shallow depth of penetration (0.3 mm). Small thermal necrosis zones provide better surgical precision and adequate hemostasis in very sensitive anatomical regions. This wavelength of laser energy is provided in slow pulse rates and therefore is inappropriate for general incisional uses. The acoustical energy of the holmium laser can provide energy for lithotripsy of gallstones or urologic calculi disruption via a photodisruptive effect. Up to three hours may be required to complete photodisruption of stones. The use of holmium lasers in this field for veterinary medicine is still investigational.

Excimer Lasers

The 193 nm excimer laser has the ability to incise tissue and leave a peripheral thermal event of less than 1 µm. The incision heals rapidly and there is minimal inflammation. This type of wavelength can actually break the C-C bonds within tissue without causing water vaporization. This is a photodecomposition effect And it has rendered the excimer laser superior for corneal refractive sculpting. This wavelength is currently in high demand for use in radial keratotomy. However, it is ineffective in a blood-filled field. Currently, cost, size, and safety considerations provide too many disadvantages for inclusion in the average veterinary practice.

Evolution of Laser Technology Advancement

Because CO_2 and diode laser energy are the primary types of wavelengths currently in use by the general veterinary community, these units will be considered more closely in this discussion.

Be aware that there are two types of CO_2 lasers on the market today: DC (direct current electrical) excited and RF (radio frequency) excited. The purpose of the excitation is to drive the CO_2 molecules into high-energy states from which laser light (photons) may be extracted. How the electric current is delivered differentiates the newer RF excited gas slab technology introduced in 1991 from the older glass tube DC excited technology introduced in the early 1980s. Glass tube DC excited lasers were originally called flow through because they required periodic re-charging of the gas mixture. This technology was updated in 1990 to a sealed tube configuration that did not require re-charging. In a DC excited laser, an electric DC current is passed through a gas-filled glass tube, producing photon excitation. In a RF excited laser an electric current is passed through a given number of inert metal plates separated by a small slab of gas, producing ionized molecules and a laser beam. RF excited lasers are often referred to as pulsed lasers while DC excited lasers are referred to as continuous wave lasers. This is not to be confused with the continuous wave mode of the laser in which the laser beam is on continuously when the laser is activated. All CO_2 lasers provide a pulsed mode. This is commonly referred to as superpulse, ultra pulse, nova pulse, sharp pulse or surgi pulse, depending on the manufacturer. From a cost standpoint, RF technology is more expensive than DC technology but RF technology tends to have a longer life cycle and is capable of producing higher pulsed energy output. The current active life cycle estimates are approximately 10,000 hours for DC excited lasers and 45,000 hours for RF excited lasers.

Delivery Systems

There are currently three primary methods of delivering laser energy from the laser chassis to the operative site: articulated arm; hollow wave-guide; and various silicone, quartz, or low OH optical transmitting fibers. A fourth delivery system incorporating a flexible enhanced transfer wave-guide that can fit into endoscopic ports is receiving final FDA approval.

CO_2 lasers employ either the articulated arm or the hollow wave guide, whereas diode, Nd:YAG, argon, and holmium lasers are delivered by an optical fiber which conducts the laser beam through reflection or refraction to the operative site. Optical fiber delivery is primarily used in endoscopic procedures in an aqueous environment where CO_2 is not applicable because it is absorbed by water.

The type of laser energy used will have a direct bearing on the guiding medium. It is critical to understand which type of laser energy is being demonstrated. Each type of laser energy interacts with the target tissues differently. Quartz optical fibers are used by laser energy that can be transferred by this medium. Diode laser energy is transferred by this type fiber. Drawbacks to these fibers are that they can become cracked or damaged and thus reduce the capacity to carry laser energy. The end also has to be renewed (cleaved) each time the laser is reused. Sterilization of the tip can also be an issue. Fibers are, however, the least expensive delivery media. Advantages to this type of delivery system come from the enhanced ability to transfer laser energy through fibroscopic devices for use deep inside body structures.

Articulated arms deliver the laser beam by means of sets of mirrors down the length of hollow composite tubes articulated and hinged to provide flexibility of movement. Hollow wave-guides transmit the laser beam down the lumen of the flexible guide by reflection of its polished surface.

Articulated arms transmit the laser beam with minimal power loss and maintain beam coherence. They also can transmit high power levels of CO_2 energy to the target tissue. However, they can be cumbersome to use. The mirrors can also cloud or become misaligned over time. This can require off-site servicing and be costly and they are not always easy to change out. Most articulated arms are less positional, especially when working in the oral cavity or ear, and require more care when handling.

Flexible wave-guides are more versatile in restricted areas. They allow for easier maneuvering of the hand piece intra-operatively. They have a greater power loss from proximal to distal end that has to be made up by increasing the joules of energy being emitted from the housing. Hollow-wave guides are considered by many to be the latest technological advance and they afford a mirrored inner surface through a flexible transport device for the laser energy. These devices are very maneuverable and positioning is often more natural. The greater advantage of this delivery system is the ability to exchange a failed or damaged one for an operating one in the clinic without special technical support and a minimal time requirement. The per unit cost of these delivery systems is also less than articulated arm transmission systems.

Each delivery system has benefits and drawbacks, which the user should weigh before determining which will provide the best application for its intended use. No one delivery system is optimal 100% of the time. The user must consider which one will provide the most consistent positive application effect. Until dual delivery systems are available, there will likely be a need for both reflective transmission and optical fiber conduction of laser energy.

Age of Equipment

It is always preferable, in our opinion, to have the most advanced technology available. In selecting lasers, there is the potential that a new laser may in fact be old technology that has just not been sold yet. This may particularly be the case with foreign manufactured lasers. While they may have never been fired, their component parts may not be state of the art and may in fact be outdated or have degraded with time in storage. A major point of consideration to help determine the technical age of a laser is the type of device that contains the molecules that emit the photons, and the type of energy used to stimulate the molecules.

The most current technology uses an RF excited laser medium. A radio frequency is passed through a given number of inert metal plates separated by a small slab of gas, producing ionized molecules and a laser beam. The radio frequency wave allows for minimal creation of heat in the chamber and tube, which in turn allows for use of simpler passive cooling of the unit that does not require refilling, pumping, or repair. This also reduces wear and tear on the internal hardware or failure in systems that have no monitoring of cooling fluid levels.

Older technology uses steel or glass canisters to hold the laser-energy-producing medium and DC electrical energy to excite the molecules to emit photons. A much greater amount of heat is generated during this process. This type of technology requires active cooling via a radiator and cooling fluid passed over the canister to dissipate heat. These older systems also have O-rings at the ends of the canisters that continually expand and contract during the heating. These O-rings can eventually crack, permitting the molecules inside the canister to leak out.

Newer laser devices use power calibration chambers that give accurate readings of the actual energy output from the tip of the laser hand piece. This better assures the user that the correct power density is being achieved. The operator without technical support can also do this calibration. Sharing of techniques is also more accurate when this type of equipment power calibration is available.

Laser Beam Directors (Focusing Hand Pieces or Spot Tips):

Articulated arm lasers use a device known as a *focusing hand piece* to control the delivery of the laser beam to the targeted tissue. There are two types of hand pieces used with modern lasers, collimated and focusing. A collimated hand piece provides the same power density whether one inch from tissue or 100 feet from tissue, while a focusing hand piece has a lens- or spot-size-limiting tip that is set to focus the beam at a given optimal focal working distance. Unlike a collimated hand piece, the greater the distance from the optimal focal target distance you move the focusing hand piece, the more divergent the laser beam and thus the less the power density becomes. As the laser beam divergence doubles, the power density decreases four fold. This difference between collimated and focusing hand pieces is critical when going from cutting to ablation or contracture to heating of tissue without the necessity of changing hand pieces.

The one drawback of lens-type hand pieces is that the hand piece itself can be sterilized only under gas. Their advantage is that a significantly higher total energy can be focused through them to the target tissue. Flexible wave guide delivery systems employ a hand piece to hold the wave guide's distal end. These hand pieces act like a focusing hand piece, but have no lens to contend with; instead special tips can be inserted into the end of the hand piece. These tips allow for a variety of focal points and focal diameters of the laser beam. This allows for a multitude of clinical applications. These hand pieces and tips can be autoclaved or gas sterilized repeatedly. They can also be easily interchanged intra-operatively without loss of sterile field.

Chassis Consideration for the System Components:

Here again, there are a variety of styles of outer cases for lasers. They range from large stationary cabinet chassis to tabletop models or roller based-pedestal mobile units. Each clinician must consider which style will allow for the greatest flexibility during operation and use in their facility. In many cases, the size of the laser also depends on the power output. Low power outputs in the 10 watt to 15 watt range can be housed in a tabletop configuration or small stand-alone unit. Lasers in the 20 watt to 40 watt range are free-standing in a housing that takes up approximately one square foot of floor space and stands three feet tall. Higher-powered lasers upwards of 100 watts can take up as much as five square feet of floor space and seven feet in height. Each user must determine what power and size best suits his or her practice. The advent of the CO_2 laser, with its peak water absorption and enhanced super pulsing capabilities, has allowed lower power with exceptional vaporization and ablative potential.

The ease of transportation for use in different locations within the hospital and at remote sites may also be a consideration. Older lasers usually require more space to house their components' internal or external cooling systems. Due to the larger number of moving parts, mobility can be an issue and breakdown a greater risk. The least number of moving parts usually allows for the greatest mobility and durability. The smaller footprint and weight in the smallest chassis optimizes technician handling in a multiple-parameter usage. Diode chassis of the more current models are very small and portable. The all solid-state make-up of these laser devices, along with their small size, provides for excellent use in ambulatory situations and small spaces. They are also easily paired with fibroscopic equipment on the same table or platform.

User Interface Panels

All lasers manufactured over the past ten years have incorporated menu-driven touch panels with digital readouts. Because these systems are controlled by computer software they are very user friendly and provide a number of pre-programmed features permitting the user to customize protocols or access pre-set protocols from a database. This allows the user to rapidly modify the laser energy output, power setting, and type of beam output and geometry without significant recalculation or time spent resetting power parameters. These panels are also flat and without knobs or switches that can be difficult to handle under sterile conditions. A sterile transparent plastic cover can easily be placed over the flat pressure-sensitive push plates for use in sterile fields. These panels can also be changed out and upgraded as warranted. The most current computer hardware and software usually support units with this type of user interface. Older units may have dials or switches that require the assistance of a surgical aid or technician, should laser parameters need to be altered intra-operatively. Be sure that you and your staff are comfortable with the laser interface before committing to a specific unit.

Service Contracts and Upgrading Equipment

It is important that the laser unit's manufacturer provide a long warranty period (at least one year and optimally three years). This should cover the entire base unit, energy transfer apparatus, and focusing device. Warranties provided by dealers are less advantageous since a secondary market dealer may go out of business, leaving you without recourse or support. Rapid 24-hour turn-a-round of a defective unit should also be expected so that valuable income-generating time is not lost. Available 24/7/365 tech support should also be included. Extended warranties after the initial new coverage period and upgrades and trade-in positions for up-line devices are also advantageous when considering laser equipment.

Any used equipment that is being considered should have been re-certified by the manufacturer or a certified repair organization. It should have passed the same standards for use as a new unit. The purchaser should be able to get an extended warranty and be allowed upgrade opportunities just as with a new unit. It is critical that the history of the unit be available and certified before purchase. Without these guarantees there is no way to know how many hours of active lasing time are still available from the unit or if the components are operating properly. Most importantly, there is no way to know how much of the laser photon-producing medium inside the machine is still present or how secure it is.

Whether new or used, the purchase of a laser is a big step for the veterinary practitioner and should be considered if possible from more than a cost perspective. A company that has an extended history in the laser industry and a proven reputation for quality and reliability should optimally have manufactured the laser you are contemplating for purchase or have a long-term agreement with the manufacturer. The seller/dealer should have a track record for service and clinical support. The seller/dealer should be part of a company that will stand behind the units it sells or re-certifies, even if the person selling you the laser leaves their employment. Today there are several companies within the industry that have a good track record on service or support. Whether you are basing your purchase on price, performance, support, or a combination of all three, it is imperative that you research the company and get references from current users. Companies that sell on low price primarily may leave you with little recourse should problems occur.

These factors also should apply when purchasing a used laser that does not have a documented history and has not been re-certified by the original manufacturer. Used lasers may have been refurbished with other than OEM (original equipment manufacturer) parts. Some off-brand parts may be of inferior quality, which may potentially fail long before the OEM parts.

All individuals that you interact with during the purchase process of a laser unit should have complete working knowledge of the equipment and the company that made the equipment. They should be able to provide you with technical specifications and support material for the laser equipment you are considering. Companies should provide opportunity for hands-on educational programs or be affiliated with organizations such as the Veterinary Surgical Laser Society (VSLS) or the American Society for Laser Medicine and Surgery (ASLMS) that can provide educational opportunities. Set-up and staff training should be included in the purchase price. Full documentation and usage and safety manuals should definitely be provided. All areas of use and safety with OSHA specifications should be provided or explained before purchase. All accessory items needed for normal operations should also be provided at the time of in-servicing of the laser equipment.

Clearly, there is a lot to consider when determining the right type of laser unit for your hospital. While low prices are always appealing for used or supposedly "new" equipment, there are varieties of pitfalls that can leave that great deal gathering dust in the corner. Even worse, your experience with laser energy could lead to unwanted negative therapeutic or surgical outcomes resulting in complications for your patients and yourself. To afford yourself the best medical and surgical outcomes when using laser technology, it is critically important to know the equipment you are purchasing. You must also have a full working knowledge of the wavelength that the equipment produces. Don't be afraid to ask questions about any and all of the previously discussed criteria. Make a checklist of your particular laser priorities and compare each laser for the best fit to your practice style. If the dealer you are considering purchasing from does not know the answer, make sure he or she knows how you can get the answer before you sign on the dotted line. Ask to have the equipment demonstrated in your hospital under real operational settings.

The VSLS highly recommends that any veterinarian considering the implementation of laser energy in their surgical and therapeutic treatments take a basic course on physics, safety, equipment operations, and technique. Advanced courses are offered by VSLS, ASLMS, and at major conventions for veterinarians. These lectures can benefit practitioners who have some current experience and would like to refine their technique as well as new users.

The VSLS has just completed plans to implement a certification process for its membership that will provide additional competency in a variety of laser wavelength studies and practices.

Last, be sure that the laser equipment you are considering has a manufacturer's address, phone number, product number, and serial number. The salesperson should provide you with a technical services hotline or direct phone number. You should be able to find out everything there is to know about that machine before you purchase it. Your enhanced professional image depends on understanding how to work with laser energy. Your personal enjoyment of the laser device depends on having excellent technology and reliable support.

Part II
PRACTICAL
LASER SURGERY

Chapter 6
Safety Considerations

Surgical lasers are powerful and potentially dangerous instruments that should be used with safety and respect. Misuse can result in severe injury to the patient, operator, and support staff. However, in the hands of a trained veterinarian, the CO_2 laser is as safe today as a scalpel blade. Therefore, safety training on laser use should be mandatory.

A thorough understanding of the type of laser that you are using (Chapter 5) is vital to any discussion of laser energy. For instance, there are critical differences in spot size between the currently available hand-held laser units, which leads to marked differences in power densities. The lasers available today embody both older, well-established systems and wavelengths, and newer, cutting-edge technologies. There is no reason for clinicians to not gain the knowledge needed to handle and use laser energy.

Two of the definitive documents on the safe and effective use of laser energy in medicine are the American National Standards Institutes (ANSI) publications ANSI 136.3 and ANSI 136.1, which use standards agreed upon by the industry. Both OSHA and the Canadian Ministry of Health use very similar criteria for appropriate safety considerations. A growing body of information is available from a host of other publications. Recommended readings are included in the back of this text and should be consulted before a laser in your hands is ever applied to a patient for therapeutic purposes.

Those who have questions about the proper safety requirements for their specific lasers should refer to the owner's manual or consult the most current version of the ANSI documents. Routine use of general common sense by the clinician and staff yields the greatest positive outcomes when using laser energy. Check your system each time before you begin any surgical case.

Do not underestimate the value of designating a "laser technician" or "laser safety officer"(one person can do both jobs) to provide day-to-day operational support for your particular laser. A fully informed and competent laser technician can ensure the laser is functioning properly. Your technicians should be versed in the day-to-day operations of the laser. At a minimum, they should be introduced to the technology by the manufacture's representative at time of installation. Consider offering your technicians the opportunity to attend continuing education courses on lasers in veterinary medicine. This will give you greater consistency in therapeutic outcomes, reduce the likelihood for improper treatment outcomes due to improper equipment preparation, and limit any down time due to system failure or malfunctions. Intra-operative stresses on the clinician and staff due to equipment malfunction can lead to inappropriate surgical compromise or worse. A knowledgeable and well-trained surgical laser assistant is invaluable. Such assistance not only facilitates the surgical procedure but enhances the safety level, as well.

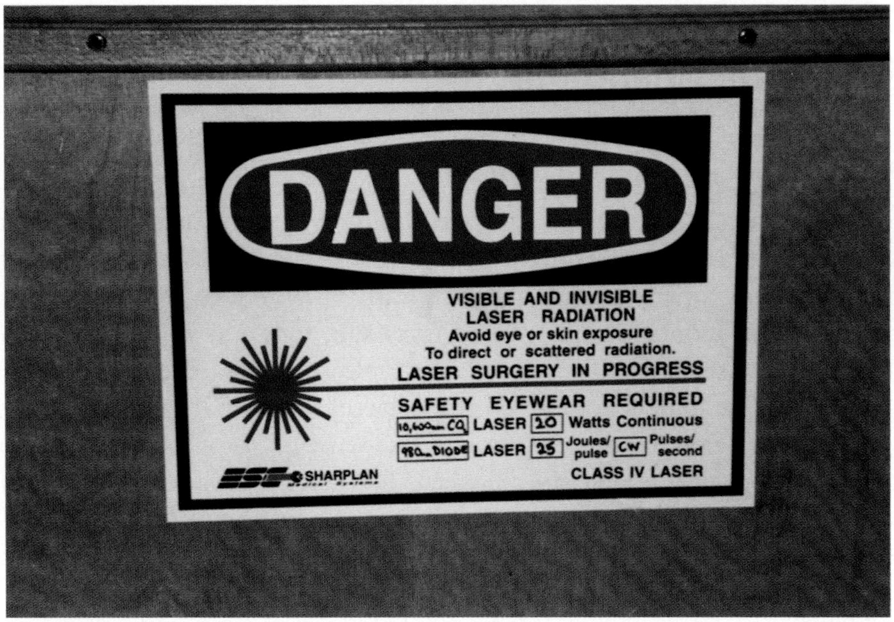

Figure 6-1 Laser identification placard showing wavelength(s) being used in the surgical room.

The laser technician can, and in most cases should, also be the "laser safety officer." This person is responsible for the administrative considerations that OSHA requires nationally and that each state may impose individually. He or she should have a working knowledge of the location of all OSHA-required support equipment and documentation prior to the laser being turned on. Some states require a radiology safety division to oversee proper laser handling and monitoring. This is true in Maryland, where one of the authors (Dr. Eeg) practices. Some states also require licensing of the laser wavelength being used. These regulations are more administrative than educational. It is the veterinary surgeon's responsibility to be aware of the potentials for injury to the assistant as well as him- or herself. (Figure 6-1) Such injury generally involves fingers holding and retracting tissues and results from improper beam positioning or reflection off of polished metallic instruments used in the procedure.

Finally, by incorporating all that you have learned into a comprehensive "to do list" that is consulted each time laser energy is used, you will avoid or greatly limit unwanted complications to the equipment, the staff, yourself, and most importantly the patient.

General Safety Guidelines

Everyone in the surgical or therapeutic room should have a working knowledge of the potential interaction between laser energy and the materials and tissues that are present.

The surgeon should only operate one foot pedal, the laser switch, in an on or off fashion. A technician should be responsible for the standby position of the laser whenever it is not in active use. The surgeon and the technician should have a clear understanding of specific requests for laser-on and laser-standby orders. In each case the laser energy components should be preset by the clinician or relayed from the clinician to the technician.

Confusion with other pedals that may be on other equipment may occur and lead to accidental firing of the laser beam and thus to inappropriate tissue, causing injury. It is critical that the veterinary surgeon be responsible for only the on/off laser foot switch. When multiple lasers are being used along with videoscopic equipment or electrocautery, the technician should place the foot pedals in the same location for each procedure or change foot pedals as requested by the surgeon during the procedure. A superior plan would be to allow the technician to control all other foot pedals, allowing the surgeon to focus on laser energy use. Multiple foot activation pedals should never be taped or bolted together. The veterinary surgeon must consciously seek out the pedal for initiation of laser energy after verbally indicating that this is the intent (by requesting laser-on status from the technician).

Plume Control

Proper and thorough evacuation of the laser plume, a gaseous and particulate byproduct of laser energy/tissue interaction, is critically important. The plume must be evacuated using approved suction devices, and protocols for when the plume evacuation system is in operation should be standard. It is critical that the technician be fully versed in the operation and implementation of plume evacuation prior to any use of a surgical laser (Figures 6-2A and 6-2B).

Although laser energy provides a high temperature environment at the point of laser/tissue interaction, viable organic material exists in the plume. The inhalation of this organic material or byproduct chemical materials left from surgical site preparation may lead to short-term or long-

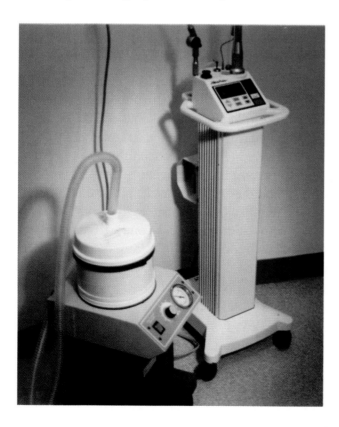

Figure 6-2A Plume evacuator (S.A.F.E. system™, Edge Systems Inc.) positioned next to 20 watt CO_2 laser (Novapulse™, Accuvet-Lumenis Inc.).

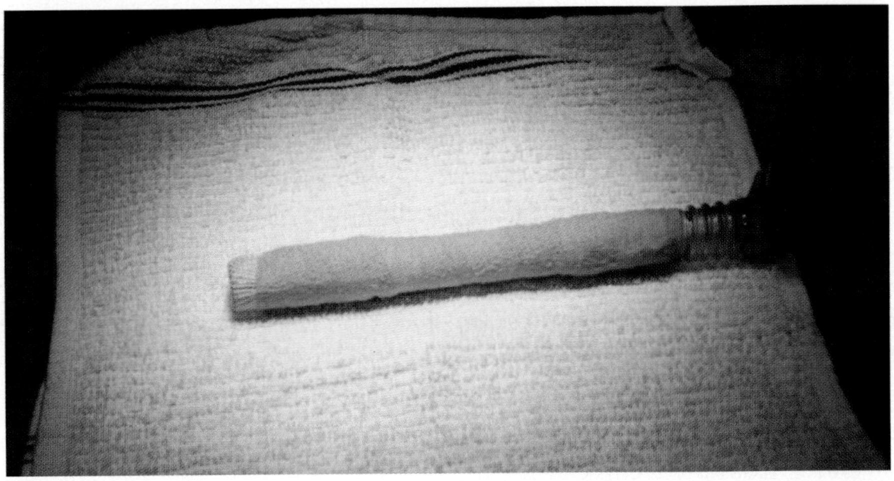

Figure 6-2B Plume evacuation handpiece prepped for use in sterile surgery field.

term respiratory irritation, damage, or disease. Please note that this is true for any component that produces smoke or a plume from its functional interaction with tissue. Electrocautery devices should carry the same requirement due to their production of smoke from the surgical site.

The laser plume creates a potential for a biohazard not only to the surgeon but also to personnel in the surgical operating room or area where laser/tissue interaction takes place. Care must be taken when the laser is used in the oral cavity or around the head so that the patient avoids inhalation of the plume. The effective use of a plume evacuator by the technical staff will reduce or eliminate the potential for hazardous inhalation. Specific plume-safe masks that have a smaller pore size (down to 0.1 um) provide further protection due to their higher filtration rate, as compared to standard surgical face masks.

Safety Considerations Regarding the Laser Unit

Both the surgeon and technician should be thoroughly familiar with the operation and care of the laser hardware and software unit. Many different laser units and wavelengths are available and the dials and scales may differ, although the underlying physics are the same. Delivery of laser energy can differ and have altering effects on the beam geometry and tissue spot interaction. Surgeons and technicians must read and understand the manual accompanying the specific wavelength and unit. Surgeons should always use new equipment in routine, well-documented cases in which they are familiar with and have great comfort with the procedure. This gives the clinician an opportunity to determine if variance in the new equipment must be factored into the tissue/laser interaction, specific safety requirements not previously considered, or physical requirements of the specific wavelength and unit.

Potential Laser Safety Hazards

The use of lasers in the clinical setting can present many hazards to the laser operator and nearby personnel. These hazards have been grouped into several classes, each of which is addressed below. This is by no means an exhaustive explanation of all potential safety issues. It is designed to provide the clinician with a starting point from which to understand what to consider when providing safety for themselves, their staff, the clients, and the patients.

Fire Hazards

High-power lasers, particularly infrared lasers (e.g. CO_2, diode, and Nd:YAG), can produce combustion of tissue, surgical gowns, anesthetic gases, tongue depressors, etc. Smoke arising from laser-induced combustion can obscure vision, and may dangerously scatter the laser beam. Therefore, preparation with wetted gauze and sterile water or saline is important to reduce the potential for injury. Attention to the surgical site will reduce or eliminate the potential for adverse outcomes. Use of high proof alcohol on the surgical or therapeutic site could cause a combustible situation and endanger the clinician, staff, and patient. Remember that OSHA requirements mandate that a fire extinguisher must be in the room where laser energy is being used.

Potential Damage to the Eyes

Accidental or intentional irradiation of the exposed eye via direct, reflected, or scattered laser light can result in damage to the cornea, conjunctiva, iris, and retina. Damage to the eyes can result in lost or impaired vision that may persist for days or longer, and can lead to permanent vision loss. Direct and reflected laser beam exposure by wavelengths between 400 nm and 1,400 nm may cause ocular transmission hazards. Corneal and lens-focusing effects increase the power density at the level of retina by five orders of magnitude. Chronic exposure may result in cataract formation or degradation of the corneal surface, iris, lens, or retina. Again, a good working knowledge of the laser/tissue interaction and the specific wavelength of laser being used will forestall the potential for ocular injury or unseen hazards from the laser energy. (Figure 6-3)

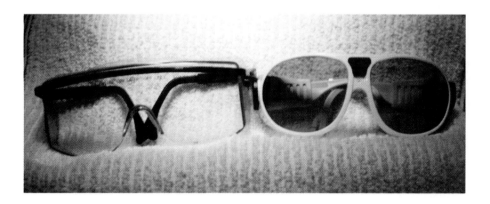

Figure 6-3 Safety glasses for 10,600 nm wavelength (L). Safety glasses for multi-wavelength use (OD 5+ @ 190 nm to 375 nm, OD 5+ @900 nm to 1,070 nm, OD 6+ @ 1,064 nm, OD 6+ @ 10,600 nm (R)).

Potential Damage to Exposed Skin

Laser irradiation of exposed skin can result in severe burns when high-power lasers are used. Long-term exposure to medium- and low-power lasers can lead to sunburn-like symptoms. It is critical that the clinician and technician understand the potential impact of a misdirected or reflected beam on skin. Laser energy can be produced from the UV to IR regions of the light spectrum, and each has its own potential for skin damage. The best defense is to actively secure the laser beam away from exposed skin surfaces not being targeted for treatment.

Electrical Hazards

Many lasers use high-voltage power supplies that can be hazardous to employees and laser operators. Only trained, certified mechanical technicians should be consulted or allowed to evaluate and repair damaged instruments. Never consider opening the housing of a laser, even if the power is turned off. Residual electrical capacity may be present and could discharge, creating a shock hazard. Lasers are electrical devices and thus must be respected for their potential to cause harm if used or handled inappropriately. Remember that 110 or 220 electrical current can pose a potential life-threatening reaction if improperly handled. Never consider operating a laser in a very wet environment where electrical conduction and discharge could take place.

Chemical Hazards

Toxic chemical hazards may exist from organic solvents that interact with or are altered by the laser energy. Coolant gases or liquids in older radiator cooled units also present potential dangers. Laser cavity byproducts (i.e., excimer lasers) are sometimes produced and can be toxic if inhaled. Photochemical reactions may occur within laser-irradiated material that escapes in the plume and is not contained in the plume evacuation unit. High-proof alcohol (200 grain alcohol) used for cleaning or sterilization can potentially be volatilized without ignition. Conversely, pure grain alcohol can be a combustible agent causing burns to the patient, surgeon, technical staff, or all three. Isopropyl alcohol can be combustible in a vapor state with adequate oxygen. To avoid this adverse reaction, flush the sterile field with sterile 0.9% NaCl prior to initiating a surgical laser beam. Oxygen acts as a strong accelerant for fire. It is critical to observe safe lasing procedures when near the endotracheal tube in the thorax. Iodinated surgical preps can be forced into the vapor state following laser exposure. Iodine vapor is extremely toxic and should not be inhaled through a surgical mask. This potential danger can be mitigated by keeping the field rinsed with sterile 0.9% NaCl and keeping it moist.

Biological Hazards

The laser plume can have components that are irritating or injurious to the mucous membranes. The respiratory tract may also be at risk for in-

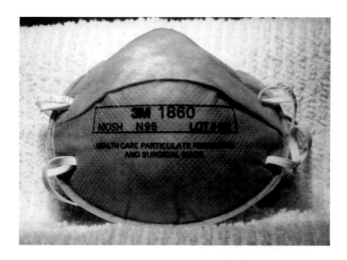

Figure 6-4 High filtration particulate respirator and surgical mask (3M Corp.).

fection, irritation, allergic reaction, or long-term debilitating effects of small particulate inhalation. Some bacterial, viral, or fungal organisms can survive in the plume. Components of the chemicals in and on the patient can be altered to become carcinogenic and potentially damaging. These components can also be drawn up into the plume. Proper plume evacuation and appropriate surgical masks (Figure 6-4) can reduce the potential for injurious long-term plume effects.

Patient Protection

A key consideration of patient protection is that anesthetized animals do not have pain reflexes. They cannot respond or move away from noxious odors or painful stimuli. The laser-producing devices and the laser energy itself use heat to work on the target tissue and produce heat as a by-product. Therefore, it is imperative that the clinician and the staff be aware of what is required to avoid the potential for injury to the patient during procedures. It is also important to remember that varying wavelengths of laser energy interact differently with tissues depending on the pigments present.

Protect eyes by using backstop titanium rods, quartz rods, saline-soaked tongue depressors, or saline-soaked gauze sponges. Ophthalmic lube protection can also be considered if the wavelength that is being used is highly absorbed by water and as an additional protectant for the cornea. Tooth enamel can also be protected in this way. Periosteal elevators can serve as backstops for procedures performed in the oral cavity.

Anodized or florentined surgical instruments can reduce light reflection by scattering an incident beam of laser light. (Figure 6-5A) The surgical instruments shown in Figure 6-5B are highly reflective and may pose a laser beam reflection hazard to the patient, surgeon, or technical staff.

Moist packing such as sterile, fluid-soaked gauze or lap sponges surrounding tissue structures can reduce or eliminate peripheral tissue injury and decrease thermal relaxation time. Protect against ignition of intestinal gases, bowel gases, anesthetic gases within endotracheal tubes, and vapors from surgical preparation solutions by always being aware of your surgi-

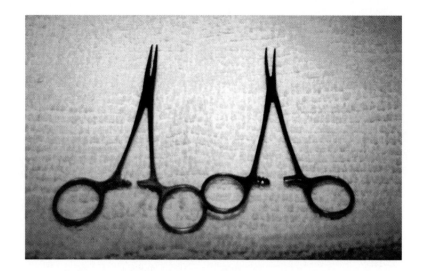

Figure 6-5A Anodized mosquito forceps used with laser surgical resection techniques.

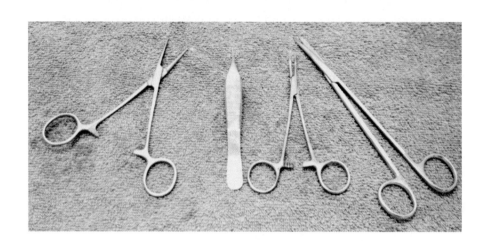

Figure 6-5B Standard reflective stainless steel surgical instruments common to most surgical packs.

cal orientation and the direction of the laser energy. Plume evacuation must always be considered, not only for the clinician and the staff but also for the patient, especially when working in the oral cavity, abdominal cavity, thoracic cavity, or in close quarters in the surgical operatory. Planned emergency procedures should always be posted in the surgery or a common area for review by staff and veterinarians at any time. Trained personnel who understand the basic issues related to laser safety must be in place before lasing commences. Safety monitoring should occur at all times, with the staff permitted to make recommendations and comment on any issues of safety that might occur.

Laser Classification

Lasers are divided into four classes according to the degree of hazard they present to humans. Grocery store scanners are termed class I lasers; they do not emit levels of optical radiation above exposure limits for the eye under any circumstances and are no more harmful than an electric light bulb. Class II lasers are best exemplified by the laser pointer. Momentary viewing of these lasers is not considered dangerous. Class III lasers are those used at laser light shows; they may be hazardous for direct viewing. Class IV lasers include all lasers that exceed 0.5 watt average power over 0.25 seconds, or those that exceed 10 joules/cm^2. These lasers can cause serious eye and skin injuries and can set fire to many materials. Both the direct and reflected beams are hazardous to the eye.

Class I: Exempt Lasers

These very-low-power lasers with an output of a few microwatts or less in continuous wave mode have no known damage potential, even after long-term intentional viewing of the direct beam. No warning labels are required. Low-level lasers used for biostimulation do require some warnings due to the wavelength of laser energy used (diode) and its potential for eye injury.

Class II: Low-Power Lasers

Class II lasers can be hazardous to the eyes if intentionally viewed for periods of several seconds or longer. The natural pain aversion reflex will normally prevent accidental eye damage from these lasers, even with direct eye exposure. Always remember that animals under anesthesia do not have the protective reflex reactions needed to avoid pain or noxious odors. Power outputs are a few milliwatts or less in continuous wave emission. Warning labels are required.

Class III: Medium-Power Lasers

Class III lasers have the potential to damage eye tissue faster than the natural aversion reaction (less than 0.25 seconds). Diffusely scattered beams are not usually hazardous to exposed skin, but over longer periods can create discomfort or actual lesions on the skin. Class III lasers can be subdivided into two groups: class (III a) lasers, which are only hazardous to the eye when focused by an optical device (such as binoculars), and class (III b) lasers, which are hazardous even when not artificially focused. Class III lasers have output powers of 5 mw to 500 mw. Warning labels are required.

Class IV: High-Power Lasers

Most of the lasers marketed to veterinarians are in this category. An output power greater than 0.5 watts continuous wave is required for this classification. Class IV lasers present potential serious hazards to the eye and skin from accidental exposure with either direct or diffusely reflected laser light. Class III and IV lasers pose serious hazards to nearby personnel as well as to the laser surgeon. Warning signs (Figure 6-1), optical shielding, and built-in safety components to shut off the laser in an emergency may be required. A laser safety officer must be named and a log must be kept when this laser is being used clinically.

Although no mandatory training is required to use a surgical laser, there are several federal agencies that regulate health care lasers. The Center for Devices and Radiologic Health (CDRH), a branch of the Food and Drug Administration, has standardized the manufacture of laser devices and is responsible for built-in safety features such as manual and automatic shutters, warning labels, time delay standby mode, and safety interlocks (not required in veterinary medicine). OSHA has oversight authority in the area of laser devices and worker safety. Some states and local municipalities may require specific registration and licensing of operators and institutions. Always check with state agencies as to proper licensing and registration requirements.

Laser Safety Guidelines

Laser administrative controls are the best way to ensure that laser safety is maintained to adequate standards. Establishing a laser safety officer is the first step in ensuring that education, training, and safety standards are maintained. The laser safety officer's duties, according to ANSI guidelines, should include (but are not limited to) the following responsibilities:

- Classify or verify classification of laser systems
- Evaluate hazards of laser treatment areas
- Assure that the prescribed control measures are in effect and recommend or approve alternates when the primary measures are not feasible
- Approve operational procedures, including any procedural checklists
- Recommend or approve protective equipment, and assure that it is periodically inspected to ensure proper working order
- Approve wording on signs and equipment labels
- Approve installation and equipment prior to use, as well as modifications to existing equipment and facilities
- Assure adequate safety education and training is provided for all personnel

The laser safety officer often assumes the additional responsibility of keeping laser use and maintenance logs which includes:

- Laser procedure and duration
- Anesthesia protocol
- Power settings
- Accessories used
- Problems and their resolutions

Controls should be in place to guarantee that only personnel with adequate safety and usage training have access to the laser. Traffic control in the laser treatment area should be practiced during laser use. Eye protection must be available and worn in the laser treatment area, and adequate warning signs must be posted at all entrances.

Windows in the laser treatment area may need to be covered if they are within the nominal hazard zone for the laser in use. Light wavelengths between 300 nm and 4,000 nm will transmit through window glass. Window glass has an optical density of 10^5 (transmitting only 1/100,000th the original intensity) for laser wavelengths less than 300 nm and also for wavelengths greater than 4,000 nm. Window glass alone provides adequate protection against transmission of the laser energy at these wavelengths, so it need not be covered when using wavelengths within these ranges. When using laser between 300 nm and 4,000 nm, however, adequate glass coverings must be used to absorb any potential stray laser beams.

Hazards associated with laser use in veterinary medicine fall into the following categories: beam hazards and non-beam hazards. Beam hazards are associated with accidental direct and reflected eye and skin exposures. Non-beam hazards center on the production of airborne contaminants, ignition of flammable substances, and electrical components of laser systems.

Laser energy and its associated reflections represent a significant potential for serious injury to several structures of the eye. Light from some lasers can cause severe corneal or retinal damage without any accompanying pain if the laser is focused on an extremely small spot. CO_2, holmium, and erbium lasers, with their radiation in the far infrared portion of the light spectrum, affect the cornea. The light is absorbed by the corneal epithelium, resulting in burning, scarring, or opacification. For lasers in the visible and near-infrared region of 400 nm to 1,400 nm, such as argon, fd Nd:YAG, tunable dye, diode, and Nd:YAG, the main potential hazard is damage to the retina. Eye protection should be rated specifically for the laser wavelength in use. The eyewear should be labeled with the optical density and wavelength to ensure optimal protection. Eyewear should have adequate side protection, as well. Contact lenses and regular glasses without side protection do not provide adequate coverage of the eye. Eyewear must be inspected regularly for damage and replaced as indicated.

Skin is the second most vulnerable area of the body to laser hazards. The damage from direct and reflected laser light is thermal and appears as an erythematous reaction. Wearing gloves and gowns and using moist drapes and sponges offers protection from reflected laser energy. Safe handling procedures are vital to protect non-target tissue from exposure to direct laser light.

Airborne contaminants are produced within a smoke plume when tissue is vaporized. In early days, lasers were believed to have evaporated tissue to the molecular level, giving off only water and CO_2. Laser-tissue interactions actually produce a plume of smoke that may contain bacterial particles, viral particles, and chemical carcinogens. The bacteria and viral particles are small, with diameters from 0.1 to 0.3 microns. The carcinogens produced are chemicals such as benzene, formaldehyde, phenol, and toluene. Levels of these chemicals can exceed OSHA limits. A smoke evacuator should be used to protect operators against the smoke plume hazards. Special laser filter masks rated for laser use are also available. These masks are designed to filter particles of 0.2 micron and larger. Standard surgical masks do not offer protection against particles of this size.

Fire safety should be respected and practiced with lasers. Surgical drapes should be made from flame-retardant material and protected with moistened towels and sponges near the primary laser beam. Water or saline and a fire extinguisher should be readily available. The laser should not be used in the presence of flammable anesthetics, prep solutions, drying agents, petroleum ointments, or flammable plastics. Methane gas produced in the gastro-intestinal tract can also represent a fire hazard. Adequate bowel preps and the insertion of a moistened sponge in the anal opening reduce methane hazards when performing surgery in the perineal area. Fire is always a hazard in the presence of an oxygen-rich environment. Upper airway surgery should only be performed with endotracheal tubes that limit penetration by the laser light. Special "laser safe" tubes may include nonflammable metal tubes, specially wrapped red rubber tubes, or 100% silicone tubes. The endotracheal tube cuff should be filled with saline instead of air and the endotracheal tube protected with moistened sponges. Special anesthetic protocols may need to be used to reduce oxygen in the airway to further reduce combustibility.

Electrical hazards associated with laser use are addressed at the manufacturing level. Interlocks limit access to high voltage components within the laser, providing access only to trained personnel. Adequate amperage and voltage should be available to the laser system. Avoid fluids around the equipment and electrical cords to minimize possibilities of a short circuit.

Reflection hazards are always a concern when using laser energy. Laser energy is delivered to tissues by either collimated or focused laser handpieces. Collimation guides channel and deliver laser energy at a constant power density over distance. Focused laser guides condense the laser energy to a preset focal distance, resulting in an increase in power density at the focal point. The focused laser energy rapidly declines beyond the focal point, resulting in a significant drop in power density over a short distance. Collimated laser energy has a higher potential of reflection than focused laser energy due to the maintenance of beam integrity and collimation over time. Nevertheless, it is recommended that any instruments used within the vicinity of a laser beam have a non-reflective finish. Backstops should always be used when appropriate and available to protect underlying tissue from reflected laser energy.

It is essential that all personnel be trained and educated on laser physics, safety, and operation to provide a laser-safe environment for both the operators and the patient. A thorough understanding of laser wavelength and tissue interaction, potential hazards associated with laser use, and use of the recommended standards for safe operation will result in safe and successful laser applications with minimal complications.

Chapter 7

Economic Considerations for Use of Laser Energy in Veterinary Medical Practice

General and specialty veterinary practices must consider a number of important factors when considering the implementation of laser energy or investing in additional types of laser energy. In addition to the reported medical and therapeutic considerations, there are economic considerations, positioning issues, staff questions, and marketing concerns. It is not our goal to delve into whether or not individual veterinary practices should implement laser energy. We strongly believe in both the therapeutic and economic impacts that appropriate laser use can have on a veterinary practice. Previous chapters, which discussed the specifics of laser technology and types, will hopefully allow the veterinarian to determine which laser is best for their patients and practice. This chapter seeks to support the veterinarian who has determined that laser energy would be of medical and therapeutic value to the practice and who is now looking for confirmation that it is economically viable, supportable, and profitable.

The following cost-to-benefit analysis (Figure 7-1) is a simplistic form of more complicated formulas for determining roughly how a purchased piece of laser technology will or will not support itself from an economic standpoint. This simple analysis can help practitioners modify their current cost structure or caseload implementation.

For laser energy to produce a positive economic incentive, the final number should be at least zero, and more favorably, in the thousands of dollars. However, this is only focusing on the equipment aspect. Remember that all cost factors related to a positive cash flow must also be evaluated.

First and foremost, you must decide if laser surgery will be an option offered to your clients, or a required cost of your surgical case management. It is essential that you make this decision before you invest time and money on an invoicing system. We feel that it is in the best interest of the patient to require laser use when the clinician deems it necessary. This does not mean that you should not inform the client that a laser is being used and charged for. It does mean that you are committed to doing what is best for the patient and teaching the client about need and value. Ask for your staff's input on this issue. Also consider surveying your best 50 to 100 clients on their feelings about your proposed new charges for laser surgery. You may be surprised at how accepting they are of this type of new technology and the improvement in care it can provide for their pets.

Fee Structures

Be sure to create an invoicing structure that is consistent with the way you charge for other technology. This is the easiest to implement with respect

Laser Energy Economic Cost-Benefit Analysis

Annual Cost for Laser Equipment

- Final established cost of laser   _____
  (divided by)
- Life expectancy or years leased   ÷ _____
  (equals)
- Amount that equipment must generate/year   _____
  (plus)
- Miscellaneous costs, disposable, etc   + _____
  (plus)
- Lease costs, interest on loan   + _____
  (equals)
- Expected Annual Expense for Equipment   _____

Estimate of Income Generated Annually by Laser Equipment

- Number of Procedures per week   _____
  (multiplied by)
- Average laser specific charge per case   x _____
  (equals)
- Income generated per week   _____
  (multiplied by)
- Weeks of laser surgery per year   x _____
  (equals)
- Income generated by laser use per year   _____

Profit-(Loss) on Laser Equipment

- Income generated by laser use per year   _____
  (minus)
- Expected Annual Expense for equipment   − _____
  (equals)
- Net Profit or (Loss) on equipment per year _____

Figure 7-1 Profit/loss worksheet.

to the staff. There are a variety of fee generation structures that can be considered. The four main types will be reviewed here.

No additional fee: A few laser surgeons charge no additional fees for the use of a laser. They indicate that marketing and an increased number of surgical procedures generate sufficient additional funds to support the use of a laser and provide the benefits previously discussed.

Laser usage level: Another option is to determine a price per unit time that the laser is in operation. For this to be practical you must have a general knowledge of how many procedures you do annually, the average amount of time spent in surgery each year, and the total annual cost for the laser. A 30% to 40% profit margin for the use of the laser should also be added to the final number. Table 7-1 outlines such a laser usage level option.

This is a simple method that allows the front office staff or the technician to enter the cost of the laser use without having to discuss the relative value with you. Group specific procedures within each computer code for tracking and trending analysis.

Table 7-1 Usage level fee structure

Computer bar code	Laser on-time	Sample fee	Sample Sx
00001	5min	$45.00	skin mass
00002	15min	$75.00	OHE
00003	30min	$125.00	Abd. Sx.
00004	60min	$250.00	amputation

Table 7-2 Fee-simple structure

Computer bar code	Laser level option	Fee for option
00001	level 1	$0.00
00002	level 2	$25.00
00003	level 3	$50.00
00004	level 4	$75.00
00005	level 5	$125.00
00006	level 6	$200.00

Fee-simple laser options: This method removes the time consideration from the equation by lumping a number of different procedures into one of six option levels. Table 7-2 shows an example of such a laser fee structure.

The level assigned to each procedure should represent the extent of the laser equipment and supplies used.

Level 1 can be used for pro bono work so that the laser's use can be tracked for these nonprofit procedures. Level 6 should be reserved for extended procedures in which special additional laser components—such as a mechanical scanner or extended on-time during granuloma bed resection—are considered.

Individual surgical procedure charge: The fourth charge structure is the most time consuming to institute. It has significant advantages on the back side for accounting and management purposes. The set-up requires a separate computer bar code for each specific role the laser plays in the procedure. This requires the surgeon or surgeons and the office manager to outline the cost of the laser's use in each surgical procedure. The time requirement, supplies, unit cost of the laser, and special support technology components must be factored into a set fee. That fee is then charged as a line item on the invoice, as seen in Table 7-3.

Table 7-3 shows that procedure has its own laser fee set up in a computer bar code. The advantage lies in how specific management can be in determining both the use of the laser per case and profitability of the laser in different areas. This allows for more specific fine tuning of the fee structure to maximize the laser's profitability. The down side is that this method is more labor intensive.

Establishing an appropriate fee structure requires an understanding of all the costs that go into owning a laser, and providing for a surgical section in the practice. This can often be an excellent time to re-evaluate cur-

Table 7-3 Sample individual invoice
Invoice for "Sparky" Smith, skin mass resection

Computer bar code	Number	Supply/procedure	Cost
00120	1	Surgical room	$45.00
00201	1	Surgical supply	$35.00
00212	1	Laser fee/skin mass	$75.00
00243	20	$3.03/min Dr. 2	$60.60
00345	1	Anesthesia	$85.00
01222	1	Histopath	$125.00
12002	1	Pre-surgical lab	$37.50
20020	10	Analgesic meds	$23.50

rent cost structures within the surgical section. Get input from the staff and office management related to the computer system, expectations, and potential pitfalls with the proposed fee structure.

These types of fee structures can help practitioners avoid subsidizing the laser through other surgical costs. Each doctor has the fee responsibility removed from his or her purview, allowing for greater consistency and better fee capture per case.

Fee structuring also permits more accurate estimates of surgical procedures for clients, which can greatly improve the acceptance rate of clients to recommended procedures. It also allows the doctor or technician to explain the value-added component the laser brings to the procedure. Without question, this allows the hospital to provide the highest level of care and be appropriately compensated for such an effort.

Indirect Benefits

How do you and your staff perceive the laser's value from a non-monetary standpoint? Using this technology can give you an opportunity to educate clients about the emotional and quality-of-life aspects of your practice possibly increasing client loyalty. Will the implications of laser energy prompt clients to seek more visits, accept additional procedures, and recommend a laser-equipped practice to their friends and family? The increased traffic and caseload may offset less-than-expected laser fees generated for the practice.

Most clinicians that we have spoken with who use laser energy to enhance and augment their treatment options feel that laser energy increases their visibility among both clients and potential clients. The enhanced image, expansion of treatment options, and increased comfort to the patient are all non-specific economic factors that have shifted the standard concept of cost-to-benefit ratio with respect to income generated specifically by laser equipment.

The staff's impression of laser use in your practice is critical to successful use and profitability. "Staff inertia" can be a significant hurdle to overcome if the laser is not first positioned correctly to the staff. We made sure to discuss and explain the value of laser energy for surgical and medical therapeutics with our staffs. We then took the additional step of provid-

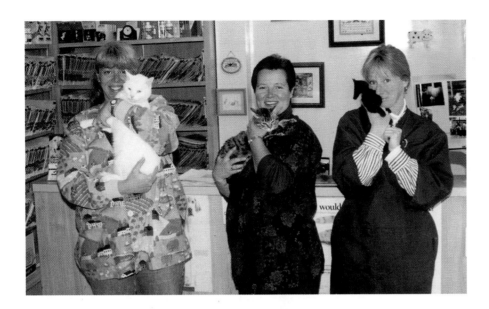

Figure 7-2 Staff members holding their personal pets following successful laser procedures.

ing surgical management to each staff member's pet for any procedure they were considering, from a simple lumpectomy to more involved routine procedures. The staff members were empowered to evaluate their pets' recovery, level of post-operative discomfort, and healing. In the end our staff members became cheerleaders for the laser, rather than detractors (Figure 7-2).

Positioning Laser Energy in Your Practice

Marketing

A number of factors affect the way people think of laser use in veterinary medicine. However, it is possible for veterinary surgeons to manage the public perception of laser veterinary surgery. From a professional perspective, veterinary practices must convey the up-to-date technical proficiency of their staffs. The appropriate use of laser energy indicates a commitment to continuing education and professional development.

In addition to staying abreast of technological advances, it may be useful to take marketing courses. This can help you think creatively about improving client communication and elevate awareness about your expertise with laser energy. Make sure your clients see the extra steps you have taken to provide a value-added service by instituting laser use. A "laser shrine" in the front office is a good way to get the word out to your clients about the value of lasers. (Figure 7-3)

Philosophy

Take a close look at the public's impressions about their animals. Although there are regional factors that affect some of these impressions, there is also a commonality in the United States about how animals are considered within the family unit. The public is more sensitive to their pet's quality of life than ever before. The public is more proactive in seek-

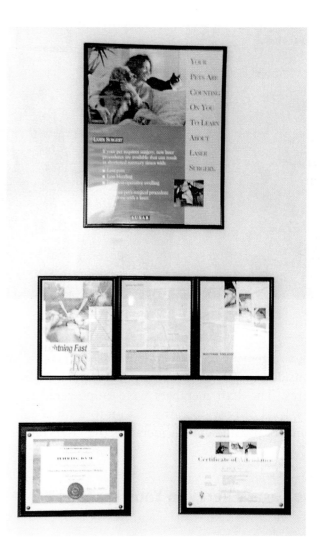

Figure 7-3 "Laser shrine" wall marketing.

ing quality veterinary care, and easy access to information is making more savvy pet owners. The expansion of the Internet is revealing itself to be a huge source of information, some good and some not so good, with respect to animals and their health needs. Chat rooms abound with individuals providing their personal impressions and recommendations. Our profession has to strive to be seen as the definitive source for any information about preventative health care and treatment for the pet-owning population. It is critical that pet owners view new technology and advances in medicine as good and important to their pets' health.

We as one of the top three caring professions in the United States, must be always ready to understand and embrace good technology and medicine. Some advances come and go but the truly profession-enhancing ones, such as laser energy, grow and enhance our reputations as quality, caring, healers for the animals we serve.

The Media's Role

The media are regarded by pet owners as a critical frontline source of information about new technology and medical advances. Although animal care is not a primary topic of media coverage, there is some subtle and some not so subtle evidences that the media are beginning to pay more attention to what the animal-owning public wants to learn about. Routinely now, you can find sections in the newspaper and general interest magazines that discuss animal health issues. Many big and small papers have a question-and-answer area for pet owners.

We would all go crazy trying to access and read all the real science and home-brewed ideas that are being circulated. But we also must realize that our clients are reading this information. We have to at least understand where pet owners get their information outside of our office. We should have a greater hand in making sure that the information they are getting is good and level. If we fail to do this we will have to spend the majority of our time putting out the small, "I read this or heard this so it must be fact," bad information fires that clients bring to us. Veterinarians and their staffs must be aggressive and proactive about providing facts to their clients and the pet-owning public.

Disseminating the Information

When we introduce our clients to the concept of laser energy, we should provide the information in a building block fashion. We can begin a continuing dialogue by packaging the information in units that can be handed out or discussed during an office visit. (Figure 7-4) These materials also can be used by the front office staff when a client requests information about a laser procedure. A technician can then be called on to provide any additional information to make the client as receptive as possible to the idea of laser surgery. This can reduce any potential "sticker shock" over the added fee structure.

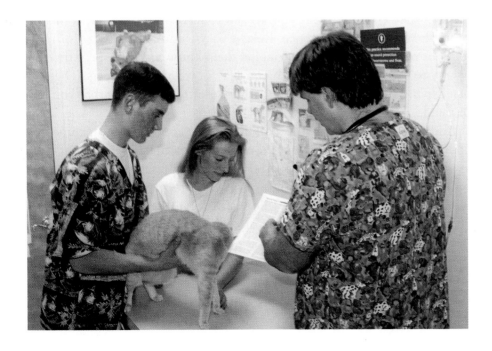

Figure 7-4 Staff and veterinarian use building-block information to discuss a potential laser surgical procedure with a client.

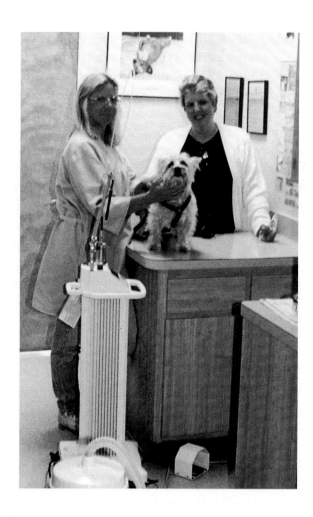

Figure 7-5 Staff member with client after a minor surgical laser procedure.

A simple introduction to the idea of laser energy from you or a staff member can set the groundwork for using a laser procedure when time arises Figure 7-5.

Take a few moments and think about how you first learned about laser energy. Then consider what you needed to feel comfortable with the idea of using lasers in your practice. Relay this to your clients in the form of a letter or personal communication. Let them know that you spent time and energy to provide them with a better way of treating their pets. Then you can expand on a case-by-case basis the uses for laser energy that you have in mind.

Additional elements of the building-block concept may include brochures, interesting case presentations, written scripts for the front office staff and technicians, and web sites. Interactive presentations are another option. We find that open houses and trips to primary and secondary schools are great opportunities to open dialogues with clients.

When writing for publications or web sites, be sure the information in general and factual. Have several of your non-veterinary friends read the information and comment on what they perceive in the piece before you run it. This can save you a lot of back peddling when misinformation is released, especially in long-running publications like the yellow pages.

Final Economic Considerations

Everyone knows that a positive income-to-expense ratio is key to the financial health of your clinic, your staff, and yourself. We have a huge responsibility to evaluate and understand new therapeutics and technology. We also have to look into our crystal balls and determine what the pet-owning public in our locale will be intrigued by or discount as unimportant. Then we have to match what will work with what we can afford, all the while realizing that other areas of revenue generation are going to decline or be eliminated for a variety of reasons, all beyond our control.

It becomes starkly evident that our professionalism, expertise, and clinical skills are what we must focus on to generate the lion's share of a stable income for our practices. Many veterinary economists have said that veterinarians who rely on product sales to generate more than 30% of their net income will place a great hardship on their ability to maintain a viable practice.

Laser energy provides a critical ability for veterinarians to maintain the professional and expertise skill level that clients require. Consider your desire to increase your surgical skills. A laser, like a scalpel, is only a surgical tool. If you are dangerous with a scalpel blade in surgery, you will be dangerous with a laser. In other words, a laser does not immediately improve the individual surgeon's skills. Superior surgical case management stems from making good, common-sense decisions and following accepted surgical practice.

Consider the impact of a positive client perception of new technology in your practice on your economic bottom line. Laser procedures can be discussed by phone, in print, and on the Internet, but your clients cannot get the services without coming to the practice.

Another factor to consider is whether you are using your other current equipment in a profitable manner. A laser by itself will not automatically be a profit center for the practice. You must have a profitability plan in place similar to your other equipment such as radiology, ultrasound, fibroscopic, in-house laboratory, and monitoring/support equipment. Before you purchase a laser, review these other professional service fee centers for adequate profitability. Then you can more easily incorporate lasers into your marketing and sales structure.

Once you recognize the need for a laser you must consider whether to lease or buy the unit. The first individual you should discuss this with is your accountant. Accountants differ in philosophy about leases, lease to buy, and purchase. Make sure you do what your accountant says. Also consider the tax ramifications when buying new equipment.

Leasing a laser avoids tying up large sums of capital at one time. There are a number of lease options and leasing companies that would love to have your account. Let your accountant and attorney review the documents before you sign your lease. Be sure you know your up-front and back-end costs. Also be sure that the tax codes (which change like the tides) support your lease decision.

A straightforward purchase will always save on the total cost. If the clinic or veterinary corporation has enough operating capital to purchase and has not exceeded new equipment spending caps, then purchasing is the best option. The money should come from asset re-allocation and not from current operating budgets or emergency bank accounts that could have hidden interest charges.

When you evaluate laser energy or ponder an expansion of laser use, you can see that the generation of income from the devices comes from your commitment to good medicine and the educational emphasis you and your staff place on client communication. This way of thinking will allow you to implement a variety of laser-type technologies as professional services that maintain or increase the profitability of the practice.

Chapter 8
Pain Management Considerations for Laser Surgery Procedures

One of the greatest advantages of laser surgery, specifically that which uses CO_2 laser energy, is less post-operative pain. Numerous anecdotal reports in veterinary literature and studies on CO_2 laser energy's effect on human nerve segments have led to a general acceptance of this benefit during and following surgery. It is important to note that from personal experience (yes, we have inadvertently lased ourselves during procedures) the initial effect on lased tissue is a significant and intense pain at the local level. This discomfort resolves within seconds of discontinuation of the beam on the tissue. No additional discomfort is noted in the near- or far-term following tissue vaporization. We therefore have a steadfast belief in the reduction of recurrent pain response when proper CO_2 laser energy is applied to a target tissue.

Clients are becoming increasingly savvy about their pets' potential for discomfort and want to be sure the pain is controlled or alleviated. Major pharmaceutical companies spend significant marketing dollars to address the public's perception of pain and pain management. These same companies also invest heavily in educating, informing, and positioning pain management to the veterinary community.

Today, veterinary medicine is still formulating a complete picture of both mediating and alleviating pain in our patients. The level of treatment varies widely from veterinary hospital to hospital and from clinician to clinician. It is clear that daily implementation of surgical pain management benefits the patient and the veterinary-client relationship. The number of practicing veterinarians consistently using some level of pain management is growing and will continue to do so as veterinarians fully realize the improvement in patient quality of life and economic veracity to the practice.

Brief Overview of Pain Physiology

Pain is defined as an unpleasant sensory or emotional experience associated with actual or potential tissue damage, or described in terms of such damage, by the International Association for the Study of Pain (IASP). The primary goal for clinicians, when managing pain, is to maximize the absence of pain sensation or, in a single word, analgesia.

Physiologic pain is a protective mechanism by the body to warn of continuing contact with potentially tissue-damaging stimuli. It is produced by stimulation of the primary nociceptors innervated by high threshold A-delta and unmyelenated C fibers.

This type of pain teaches the body to avoid these types of noxious stimuli. This mechanism is managed by a complex interaction of nociceptors; first-, second-, and third-order neurons ascending to the brain; and sen-

Brief Overview of Drug Classes

The following five major analgesic classes are used on a daily basis in our hospitals during anesthetic prep, general anesthesia, and post-operative recovery:

- **Opioids** (morphine, fentanyl [injection and patch], hydromorphone, codeine, butorphanol, and buprenorphine)

  Action: Act primarily at the pre- and post-synaptic receptors in the peripheral and central nervous systems.

  Side effects: May increase vagal tone. May cause vomiting. May produce dysphoria, especially in the feline patient.

  Contraindications: Intracranial hypertension; may increase ocular, intracranial, intra-abdominal or esophageal pressure.

  Multimodal effects: additive or synergistic analgesic effects with alpha$_2$ agonists, NSAIDs, phonothiazines, benzodiazepines, and local anesthetics. Cardiac rate reduction can also occur and should be monitored.

- **Alpha$_2$ adrenergic agonists** (xylazine, medetomidine)

  Action: Cause hyperpolarization of brain and peripheral nerve cells associated with excitatory input. Causes cells to become unresponsive to stimuli-produced analgesic and/or sedative action, depending on the location of the cell.

  Side effects: Vomiting sometimes noted. Will increase vagal tone. Will cause reduction in heart rate and may induce bradycardia. May cause transient hypertension.

  Contraindications: Same as opioids. Arterial hemorrhage or blood clotting disorders.

  Multimodal effects: Have additive and/or synergistic effects with opioids. Can prolong duration and intensity of effect. Also have additive anesthetic effects when inhalants, ketamine, barbiturates, or propofol are used to maintain anesthesia. Allow for reduced administration of these anesthetic agents.

- **NSAIDs** (carprofen, aspirin, etodolac, meloxicam, ketoprofen, flunixin meglumine, acetaminophen, coxib)

  Action: Inhibit cyclo-oxygenase enzymes, reducing the production of inflammatory prostaglandins that sensitize peripheral nociceptors.

  Side effects: Rare hepatotoxic events have been identified. Cats require much less frequent doses. Chronic liver and kidney evaluation indicated for long-term use. Some may reduce platelet aggregation. GI irritation, ulceration, or perforation.

  Contraindications: Existing liver or kidney disease. Bleeding disorders.

  Multimodal effects: Have been shown to have additive or synergistic analgesic effects with opioid agonists and potentially with alpha$_2$ agonists. May enhance corticosteroid toxicity. Are highly protein bound and therefore compete with other highly protein bound drugs, requiring increased levels of these drugs to reach therapeutic levels.

- **Local anesthetics** (lidocaine, bupivacaine, mepivacaine)

  Action: Prevent conduction of nerve impulses by inactivated closed state sodium permeability.

Side effects: High doses can cause central nervous system and cardio-vascular toxicity. Patient may experience complete loss of sensation or limb function.

Contraindications: Bupivacaine will cause cardiovascular toxicity following intravenous administration.

Multimodal effects: Can markedly reduce requirements for general anesthetics. Opioids and alpha$_2$ agonists can be used in cocktail for epidural and intra-articular anesthesia, prolonging duration of hypoalgesia.

- **Non-analgesic dissociative/sedative drugs** (ketamine, acepromazine, diazepam)

Action: Have various action potentials for dissociative/sedative induction. Do not have a direct analgesic potential in the patient. Primarily alter nerve conduction, signal generation, or signal transmission.

Side effects: Each drug must be considered individually for the specific case being managed.

Contraindications: Beta-adrenergic antagonists may cause airway constriction in cardiovascular-compromised patients or those with bronchiolar disease.

Multimodal effects: Will potentially prolong effect of direct analgesic agents given concurrently.

Please note that the combination of one or more of the above non-analgesic dissociative/sedative classes will produce sedation and immobilization of the patient, but without any true analgesic potential. If your current protocols incorporate only these types of drugs, you are not providing true analgesic support for your patient.

Preemptive and Multimodal Combinations Used in Laser Surgical Application

The following drug combinations have and are being used in both of our general clinical practices with consistently good results for analgesic support in laser surgical patients. Multimodal combinations are grouped under general surgical regions.

General Cutaneous Tissue Laser Therapy (Granuloma Resurfacing, Local Tissue Vaporization)

Pre-operative:

NSAIDs orally 48 hours prior to surgery
Carprofen, 2-4mg/kg once daily or divided BID in dog
Carprofen, 2-4mg/kg Sub-Q 30 minutes before procedure in dog
Carprofen, 1mg/kg Sub-Q 30 minutes before procedure in cat

Sedation/analgesic:

- Dog: Medetomidine, 10mg/kg and Butorphanol, 0.2 to 0.4mg/kg and Atropine, 0.04mg/kg. All can be mixed in the same syringe and given IM. Allow 5-15 minutes for sedation/analgesic effect.

- Cat: Medetomidine,10-15mg/kg and Butorphanol, 0.2 to 0.4mg/kg and Atropine, 0.04mg/kg. All can be mixed in the same syringe and given IM. Allow 5–15 minutes for sedation/analgesic effect.
- Regional analgesic/infiltrative block:
  - Dog: Bupivacaine, up to 2mg/kg using a 25-28 gauge needle to infiltrate surrounding dermis.
  - Dog: Mepivacaine, up to 5mg/kg using a 25-28 gauge needle to infiltrate surrounding dermis.
  - Cat: Bupivacaine, up to 1mg/kg using a 25-28 gauge needle to infiltrate surrounding dermis.
  - Cat: Mepivacaine, up to 2.5mg/kg using a 25-28 gauge needle to infiltrate surrounding dermis.
- Induction: Propofol, Sevoflurane, Isoflurane
- Post-operative: None

Dispensed analgesics: Oral NSAID

- Dog: Carprofen, 2-4mg/kg, orally, BID for 5 days
- Cat: Carprofen, 1mg/kg, orally every 96 hours for 1 week.

Castration, Ovariohysterectomy, or General Abdominal Procedure

Pre-operative:

NSAIDs, orally 48 hours prior to surgery
Carprofen, 2-4mg/kg once daily or divided BID in dog
Carprofen, 2-4mg/kg Sub-Q 30 minutes before procedure in dog
Carprofen, 1mg/kg Sub-Q 30 minutes before procedure in cat

Sedation/analgesic:

- Dog: Medetomidine, 10 mg/kg and Butorphanol, 0.2 to 0.4mg/kg and Atropine, 0.04mg/kg. All can be mixed in the same syringe and given IM. Allow 5-15 minutes for sedation/analgesic effect.
- Cat: Medetomidine, 10-15mg/kg and Butorphanol, 0.2 to 0.4mg/kg and Atropine, 0.04mg/kg. All can be mixed in the same syringe and given IM. Allow 5–15 minutes for sedation/analgesic effect.

Induction: Propofol, Sevoflurane, Isoflurane
Post-operative:

- Dog: Meditomidine, 1-2mg/kg and Butorphanol, 0.2mg/kg. Administered IV after extubation to prolong and enhance analgesia and recovery sedation.
- Cat: Meditomidine, 1mg/kg and Butorphanol, 0.1mg/kg IM post extubation.

Dispensed analgesics: Oral NSAID

- Dog: Carprofen, 2-4mg/kg, orally, BID for 5 days.
- Cat: Carprofen, 1mg/kg, orally every 96 hours for 1 week.
  Meloxicam liquid, 0.1mg/kg SID orally for 3 days.

General Musculoskeletal Laser Surgical Procedures (Cruciate Ligament Repair, Muscle Mass Resection, Amputation, etc.)

Pre-operative:

NSAIDs, orally 48 hours prior to surgery
Carprofen, 2-4mg/kg once daily or divided BID in dog
Carprofen, 2-4mg/kg Sub-Q 30 minutes before procedure in dog
Carprofen, 1mg/kg Sub-Q 30 minutes before procedure in cat

Sedation/analgesic:

- Dog: Medetomidine, 10mg/kg and Hydromorphone, 0.05-0.2mg/kg, and Atropine, 0.04mg/kg. All can be mixed in the same syringe and given IM. Allow 5-15 minutes for sedation/analgesic effect.
- Cat: Medetomidine, 10-15mg/kg and Hydromorphone, 0.2mg/kg, and Atropine, 0.04mg/kg. All can be mixed in the same syringe and given IM. Allow 5–15 minutes for sedation/analgesic effect.

Induction: Propofol, Sevoflurane, Isoflurane
Post-operative:

- Dog: Meditomidine, 1-2mg/kg and Hydromorphone 0.05mg/kg. Administered IV after extubation to prolong and enhance analgesia and recovery sedation.
- Cat: Meditomidine, 1mg/kg and Hydromorphone, 0.05mg/kg IM post extubation.

Dispensed analgesics:

- Oral NSAID
  - Dog: Carprofen, 2-4mg/kg, orally, BID for 5 days.
  - Cat: Carprofen, 1mg/kg, orally every 96 hours for 1 week.
- Meloxicam liquid, 0.1mg/kg SID for 3 days
- Fentanyl Patch:
  - Dog: 0.005mg/kg/hr
  - Cat: 0.005mg/kg/hr
- Buprenorphine:
  - Dog: 0.005-0.02mg/kg PO every 4-8 hours for 3 days
  - Cat: 0.005-0.015mg/kg PO every 4-8 hours for 3 days
- Codeine:
  - Dog: 1-2mg/kg PO every 8-12 hours for 3 days
  - Cat: 0.1-0.2mg/kg PO every 12 hours.

Disarticulation Procedures (Feline Onychectomy, Canine Toe Amputation)

Pre-operative:

NSAIDs, orally 48 hours prior to surgery
Carprofen, 2-4mg/kg once daily or divided BID in dog

Carprofen, 2-4mg/kg Sub-Q 30 minutes before procedure in dog
Carprofen, 1mg/kg Sub-Q 30 minutes before procedure in cat

Sedation/analgesic:

- Dog: Medetomidine, 10mg/kg and Butorphanol, 0.2 to 0.4mg/kg, and Atropine, 0.04mg/kg. All can be mixed in the same syringe and given IM. Allow 5-15 minutes for sedation/analgesic effect.
- Cat: Medetomidine, 10-15mg/kg and Butorphanol, 0.2-0.4mg/kg, and Atropine, 0.04mg/kg. All can be mixed in the same syringe and given IM. Allow 5–15 minutes for sedation/analgesic effect.

Induction: Propofol, Sevoflurane, Isoflurane
Post-operative:

- Dog: Meditomidine, 1-2mg/kg and Butorphanol, 0.2mg/kg. Administered IV after extubation to prolong and enhance analgesia and recovery sedation.
- Cat: Meditomidine, 1mg/kg and Butorphanol, 0.1mg/kg IM post extubation.
- Dog: Mepivicaine, 2-3 drops intra-incisional prior to closure.
- Cat: Mepivicaine, 1 drop intra-incisional prior to closure.

Dispensed analgesics:

- Oral NSAID
  - Dog: Carprofen, 2-4mg/kg, orally, BID for 5 days.
  - Cat: Carprofen, 1mg/kg, orally every 96 hours for 1 week.
  - Meloxicam liquid 0.1mg/kg SID for 3 days.
- Fentanyl Patch:
  - Dog: 0.005mg/kg/hr
  - Cat: 0.005mg/kg/hr
- Buprenorphine:
  - Dog: 0.005-0.02mg/kg PO every 4-8 hours for 3 days
  - Cat: 0.005-0.015mg/kg PO every 4-8 hours for 3 days
- Codeine:
  - Dog: 1-2mg/kg PO every 8-12 hours for 3 days
  - Cat: 0.1-0.2mg/kg PO every 12 hours.

We have found these analgesic techniques to work synergistically with the use of laser energy during surgery to enhance control of intra- and post-operative pain in our patients. There are a host of other individual multi-modal analgesic techniques that individual clinicians may favor outside of those presented here. It is important that veterinary medical professionals arm themselves and their staffs with the best pain management information and surgical techniques to provide for superior pain control for their patients.

Part III
CLINICAL LASER TECHNIQUE AND PROCEDURES

Chapter 9
Diode Lasers in Small Animal Veterinary Medicine

*Jeffrey R. Moll, DVM**

Diode Lasers, Physics, and Biomechanics

Generation of Diode Laser Energy

Diode lasers that are used for surgery generate laser energy via a semiconductor chip that emits energy as light (photons). The diode laser was first operated on September 16, 1962. It was developed by a team of scientists at the General Electric Research Development Center in Schenectady, New York.[1] The semiconductors used in veterinary surgical diode lasers are most commonly composed of aluminum, gallium, and arsenide, or GaAlAs. Voltage applied to the semiconductor causes an energy shift. This energy is then released as photons or laser light. The exact wavelength of the laser light depends on the operating temperature of the unit. Other factors can also influence the exact wavelength, including the concentration of the doping elements, "the driving current, and the presence of a magnetic field."[2] A schematic representation of a diode laser semiconductor is shown in Figure 9-1.

Diode lasers are the most efficient lasers in converting electrical energy to optical energy. They have already gained popularity with large-animal practitioners due to their portability and lower purchase price. The use of diode lasers in equine endoscopic surgery has been well documented.[3,4,5] Figure 9-2 illustrates three of these units, available from a number of manufacturers.

Small-animal practitioners have begun to use diode laser energy as a complement to CO_2 laser energy. With the increased use of endoscopic equipment for minimally invasive procedures, diode lasers will find an ever increasing role in small animal surgical and therapeutic practice.

Wavelength and Tissue Interactions of Diode Laser Energy

The most common surgical diode lasers used in veterinary medicine have wavelengths of 810 nm or 980 nm and have power outputs from 10 watts to 60 watts. These wavelengths are in the near infrared region of the electromagnetic spectrum. The interaction of these wavelengths is shown in Figure 9-3, which also shows that these wavelengths are preferentially absorbed by hemoglobin, oxyhemoglobin, and melanin. Diode laser energy in the 980 nm range is also absorbed by water. This may make the 980 nm a more effective excisional and dissectional tool compared to the 810

*President, ex officio, Fellow, Veterinary Surgical Laser Society, LTD

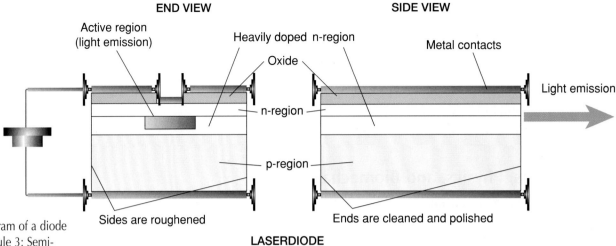

END VIEW　　　　　　　　　　　　**SIDE VIEW**

Active region
(light emission)　　　Heavily doped n-region　　　Metal contacts

Oxide　　　　　　　　　　　　　　　　　　Light emission

n-region

p-region

Sides are roughened　　　　　　Ends are cleaned and polished

LASERDIODE

Figure 9-1 Diagram of a diode laser. From Module 3: Semiconductor lasers in LEOT laser tutorial-applications in photonics and telecommunications.

nm. Water absorption of 980 nm diode laser energy is significantly lower than CO_2 laser energy.

Diode surgical lasers penetrate more deeply than CO_2 lasers. The depth of penetration of the 980 nm diode is comparable to but slightly less than Nd:YAG laser energy.[6,7] CO_2 lasers create zones of peripheral coagulation of 50 microns to 100 microns. Diode lasers create zones of peripheral coagulation of between 450 microns and 600 microns.[8] (Figure 9-4) Therefore, the underlying structures at the surgical site must be considered during treatment planning. The actual depth of significant laser tissue interaction depends on the tissue treated (thermal relaxation time), the power applied (power), the spot size (fiber diameter), the exposure time (duration), and the exposure mode (pulsed versus continuous wave).

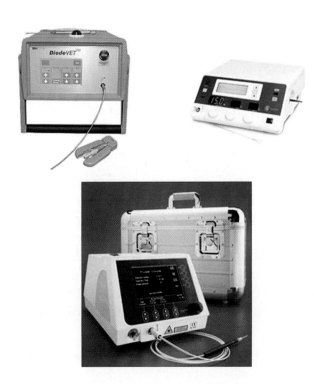

Figure 9-2 Diode lasers.

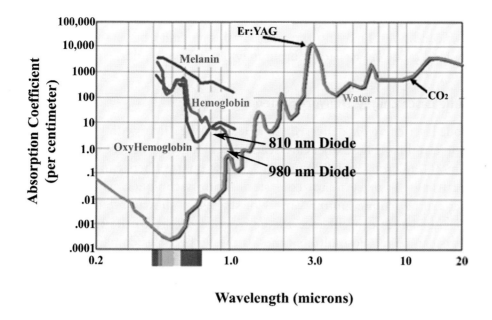

Figure 9-3 Laser wavelength absorption.

The photothermal effect of the 810 nm diode laser may be enhanced by the injection of indocyanine green (ICG) dye. Intravenous injection of this dye may allow for the more effective treatment (ablation) of skin lesions in the free-beam (non-contact) mode.[9,10] Direct treatment of the target tissue with ICG also may allow for the selective destruction of this tissue.[11,12]

Medical diode lasers are also available in wavelengths that range from 630 nm to 730 nm. These are used primarily in photodynamic therapy (PDT), which is currently being investigated in the treatment of certain neoplastic processes and chronic ulcerative tissue diseases.

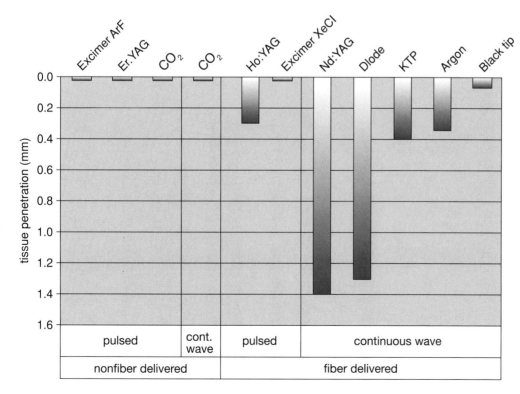

Figure 9-4 Penetration depth of different laser light in pigmented tissue.

Low-level diode laser therapy has been used to treat chronic pain and other conditions. I have no experience in this modality, but in the future this low-level diode laser energy output may prove to be clinically important.

Diode Laser Energy Delivery Systems

Diode laser energy is delivered via a flexible silica fiber with plastic or silicone cladding. These fibers are readily available in a variety of diameters from 300 microns to 1,000 microns. These quartz fibers can be re-sterilized using gas or standard cold sterilization techniques. The tip of the fiber can be sculpted into a variety of shapes, as shown in Figure 9-5.[13]

These shapes can enhance the delivery of energy to the target tissue. Fibers can be reused multiple times. If the tip becomes damaged the fiber must be replaced or reprocessed. Fibers can be reprocessed into a bare-ended fiber by stripping the plastic or silicone jacket and cleaving the tip. The tip must be cut with an instrument specifically designed for this purpose. The cleaver is usually a diamond-edged device that scores the end of the fiber, allowing it to be fractured along the score line. When reprocessing the fiber it is imperative to obtain a clean and straight cleave. This can be assessed by connecting the fiber to the laser and turning the aiming beam to medium or high. The tip of the fiber is then held perpendicular to a white background. The aiming beam should appear as a homogeneous round circle. Improper cleaving will result in this circle appearing incomplete or uneven; if this occurs, the fiber should be re-cleaved and retested. The sculpted or bare-ended tips are the most commonly used in veterinary medicine.

The fiber delivery system delivers energy through various fiberoptic and videoscopic devices. These include flexible endoscopes, otoendoscopes, laparoscopes, rhinoscopes, and cystoscopes. The delivery of laser energy through these devices has greatly enhanced the therapeutic options for the veterinary surgeon. Due to the delivery system and the wavelength, laser energy can be effectively delivered in a fluid environment. Irrigation dur-

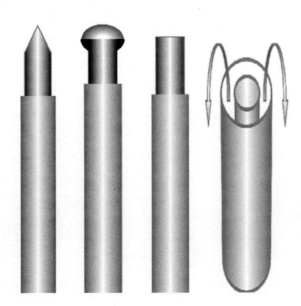

Figure 9-5 Tip shapes for diode laser fibers.

ing many of these procedures enhances visualization, controls heat, and removes treated (lased) tissue. When immersed in fluid, there is no laser plume and smoke evacuation is not required.

Handpieces allow for the use of diode fibers in general surgery. They are generally made of aluminum and can be steam sterilized in a routine fashion. A sterilized fiber is then inserted into the handpiece. Specialty handpieces with an integrated fiber are available. These allow for delivery of laser energy at various angles of up to 90 degrees (side firing) or of fixed focal lengths with spot sizes of up to 7 mm. Special air or water cooled fibers are also available; these are particularly useful in the free-beam mode. Another fiber delivery system is available with a variety of interchangeable tips.[14] These tips allow the surgeon to change the fiber tip intra-operatively to optimize the effect of the laser depending on the target tissue or whether coagulation or cutting is more desirable.

Because diode wavelengths are not in the visible spectrum, an aiming beam is used (especially in free-beam mode) to allow the clinician to properly visualize and align the target area. This aiming beam allows for the precise delivery of diode laser energy to the target tissue in the free-beam mode.

Delivery Modes

As with any laser, sufficient energy must be delivered to the target tissue to achieve the desired effect. In general terms, free-beam diode laser surgery provides for ablation or coagulation of target tissues. There are three variables that control the fluence (energy per cm^2) delivered to the tissue. They are (1) spot size, as controlled by the distance to the target and the size of the fiber (the tip diameter is inversely proportional to power density at the target tissue); (2) power, as controlled by the laser setting (watts); and (3) exposure time, as controlled by the surgeon or the laser. It is important to note that fibers rapidly begin to overheat in the free-beam mode because there is no tissue or fluid to dissipate the heat being generated at the tip. For this reason the laser exposure times must be limited when not cooled under continuous irrigation to allow for some cooling between pulses. This extends the life of the fiber tip and fiber in general.

Contact Mode: The contact mode may be used in pigmented tissues to directly deliver the laser energy to the tissue. In less pigmented tissues a thin layer of char (Figure 9-6) should be created on the tip of the fiber to enhance the delivery of thermal energy to the target. This layer of char absorbs the diode laser energy and converts it to thermal energy. The thermal energy is then directly transferred to the tissue, causing vaporization.

In the contact mode, the diode laser can be used to incise, excise, or ablate abnormal tissue. Any carbonization that occurs during the treatment process should be promptly removed by irrigation or with saline-soaked gauze sponges. Failure to remove carbonized tissue will result in this tissue absorbing the thermal energy and inadvertent collateral damage. The contact mode provides excellent hemostasis with little peripheral damage (300 μm to 600 μm).[15,16] Sterile water or isotonic saline can be used to

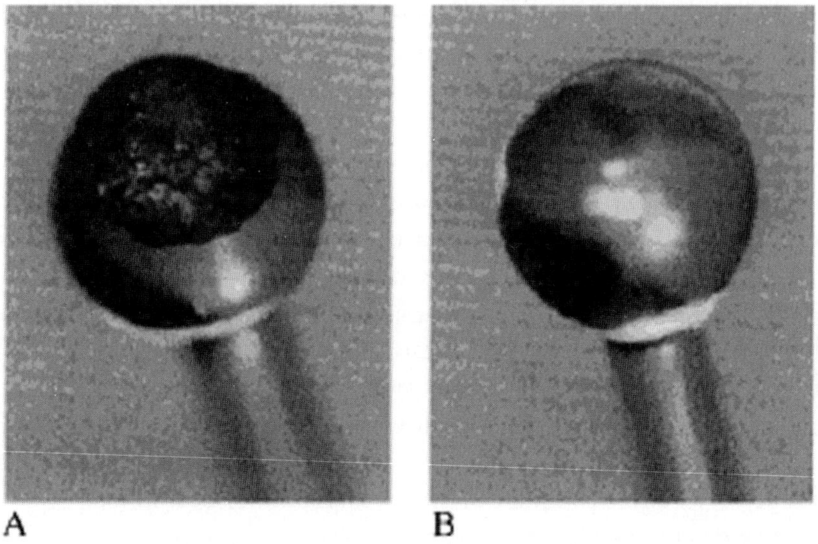

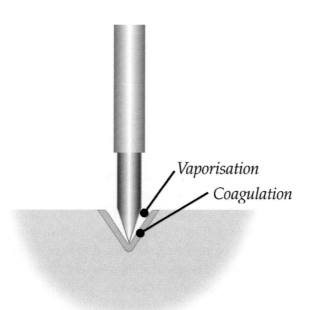

Figure 9-6 Photographs of a carbonized (A) and untreated (B) 400-micron orb-tipped laser fiber.

irrigate the target area and will help to prevent or reduce peripheral tissue damage.

At powers lower than 10 watts, the contact diode laser mode allows for excellent and precise coagulation of bleeding vessels up to 2 mm in diameter. Typically 2 watts to 5 watts will provide excellent coagulation for actively bleeding vessels. The effect of the diode laser on actively bleeding vessels is rapid and precise. The tissue interaction of the laser fiber is shown in Figure 9-7.

Free-beam Mode: In my experience the free-beam mode is practical only in highly pigmented or relatively vascular tissue. This is probably related to the power output of these lasers. Theoretically, the higher power (60 watts or more) lasers would be more effective in this mode. Free-beam ablation can provide excellent reduction in tissue that is well vascularized, either natively or due to neoplasia. This mode can be used in the 1 watt

Vaporisation

Coagulation

Figure 9-7 Laser tissue interaction; contact mode (Diomed Surgical Presentation, 1999).

to 4 watt range for photocoagulation of retinal or other ocular tissue. Effective tissue vaporization in the free-beam mode requires power outputs in the 10 watt to 60 watt continuous wave (CW) range or higher. The power required depends on the spot size. As indicated by basic laser physics, larger diameter fibers require much greater power output to provide the same power density to the tissue. The laser energy is absorbed by melanin, hemoglobin, or oxyhemoglobin in the tissue to create the desired affect. A coagulation effect on the underlying tissue of up to 3 mm can result.[17] To optimize the free-beam effect, a new fiber or a freshly cleaved fiber or one with an orb tip should be used. This reduces the amount of scatter and hence unintended peripheral damage. The maintenance of optimal power density depends on keeping the fiber tip clean and undamaged during the lasing process. The surface of the target tissue must also be kept free of any carbonization. Any carbonized material on the surface of the tissue or the tip of the fiber will absorb the diode laser energy and convert it to thermal energy. If this occurs the fiber and any endoscopic equipment may become damaged. More importantly, inadvertent peripheral thermal damage is infinitely more likely to occur. It is therefore imperative that any observed carbonized material be promptly removed. Carbonization can be reduced by limiting exposure times and irrigating between exposures. This allows both the fiber and the surface of the tissue to cool. The laser-tissue interaction is shown in Figure 9-8.

The photothermal effect of the 810 nm diode laser may be enhanced by the topical application or the intravenous administration of a chromophore (indocyanine green, ICG). This may offer the opportunity to more selectively treat neoplastic processes in the future. ICG enhances the absorption of the diode laser energy and causes selective damage to tissues containing ICG.[18] The clinical use and application of this procedure is still under development. In the future it may offer an enhanced ability to use diode laser energy more selectively in a wider variety of applications.

It cannot be overemphasized that in either mode **it is imperative to control any excess heat generated**. Failure to adequately control the heating

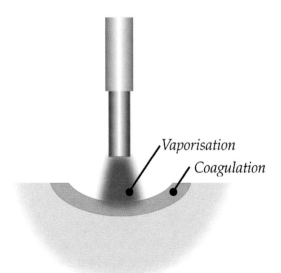

Figure 9-8 Laser tissue interaction; free-beam mode (Diomed Surgical Presentation, 1999).

of the fiber will damage the fiber, any endoscopic equipment in use, and more importantly will result in inadvertent peripheral damage. Heating may be controlled by limiting the exposure time. Exposure time may be controlled by the surgeon in the continuous wave mode. In general, exposure should be limited to less than three seconds. The laser may also be used in a pulsed mode setting to allow for tissue and fiber cooling between exposures. Exposure times can be greatly increased by irrigating the fiber and the surgical site. Regardless of the cooling method, the fiber should never appear white hot and should remain cool to the touch between exposures.

Protection of Operating Room Personnel

The standard precautions that are used with any laser are applicable and should also be used when operating the diode laser. It is imperative that safety glasses rated for use with the proper wavelength of the diode laser are employed. This is particularly important when the laser is used with fiberoptic endoscopic equipment of any type. This equipment optically magnifies the image and transmits it to the eye of the user. Any direct or indirect laser energy that is captured by the device will be directly transmitted to the user's eye. This can have severe permanent adverse consequences (retinal damage) that include loss of vision. The potential hazard is markedly reduced when a video endoscopic system is used. The image observed by the surgeon is indirect and laser light cannot cause damage. To protect the endoscopic equipment and operatory personnel, the laser should always be placed in the standby mode during insertion and removal of the fiber. Appropriate protective eyewear should also be employed during these times. Federal regulations dictate the safe use of lasers. These regulations are administered by OSHA.[19] In addition to federal regulations, twenty-six states currently have regulations regarding the safe use of lasers. Become aware of these regulations and comply with them.

The plume produced by diode laser tissue interaction can produce the same long-term health hazards as any chronic small particulate matter that is inhaled. Plume evacuation is critical. In areas where the diode laser is being used through a fiberoptic device the plume can be removed via suction from a suction tube or through the air port on the fiberoptic device. Plume will not be generated when the laser is operated in a fluid environment and in these cases plume evacuation is generally not required. There are federal regulations, and there may be state regulations, that apply to this potential hazard.[20] They should be observed to protect the surgeon and other operatory personnel.

Common Uses of the Diode Laser Energy

Conventional Surgery

Skin Incisions

Diode lasers can be used in contact mode to make routine skin incisions. In general, a sculpted or bare-end 600-micron fiber is used in a continuous wave setting with 7 watts to 9 watts of power. Because skin is a relatively avascular and non-pigmented tissue the tip of the laser fiber should be carbonized by activating the laser while in contact with a sterile wooden tongue depressor that has been marked with a black pen or indelible marker. Once this thin layer of carbon (char) has been created it is this layer that transfers the thermal energy to the tissue. Manufactured tips that have been treated to absorb diode laser energy are also available.[21] It is not necessary to carbonize these tips. It is imperative to control any excess thermal energy that may be generated in this mode. When the laser is activated without contact to the target tissue (or for prolonged periods of time) the fiber will become extremely hot. This heat can damage the plastic or silicone cladding on the fiber and cause unintentional peripheral thermal damage. This can be adequately controlled by irrigation with sterile fluid or by limiting the exposure time. Generally, exposures of less than three seconds will not result in excessive heating. This exposure time depends on the fiber diameter and the power setting (power density). It is also somewhat dependent on the thermal relaxation time of the target tissue. Pigmented skin is more easily incised than lightly or non-pigmented skin.

While skin incisions can effectively be made with the diode laser, the common diode wavelengths are not as well suited for this purpose as the carbon dioxide laser. The majority of complications are due to unintentional peripheral thermal damage by failure to adequately control the heating of the fiber. This can be adequately controlled by limiting the exposure time to less than three seconds, cooling the fiber tip in saline during or between exposures, only firing the laser when the fiber is in direct contact with the target tissue, and by removing any carbonized material from the target tissue as it occurs.

Feline Onychectomy (Declaw)

There has been much debate concerning the use of the diode laser for this procedure. Much of this controversy arises from the adverse results obtained by surgeons inexperienced with this laser. It has been my experience that the diode laser is safe and extremely effective for this procedure when proper tissue handling and thermal-tissue interaction precautions are used. The reported complications appear to stem from unintentional thermal injury. The primary reported problems have been excessive tissue swelling, tissue necrosis, and infection. In more than four years of clinical use these complications have never been encountered at my facility. Pain control, hemostasis, and post-operative healing time have been indistinguishable from the results that have been achieved with the CO_2 laser. When used in a contact mode the diode laser provides superior tactile feedback and handles much like a scalpel blade. This allows for precise dissection of the third phalanx and precise coagulation of the vascular structures (Figures 9-9 and 9-10).

The procedure is similar to that outlined above for skin incisions. Control of excess thermal energy is paramount due to the delicate nature of the tissues. It is especially important to properly carbonize (char) the

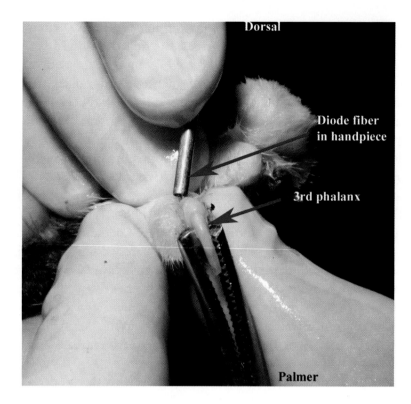

Figure 9-9 Intra-operative anterior view; feline onychetomy.

tip of the fiber. This will ensure effective and efficient transfer of thermal energy to the tissue. For this procedure a 600-micron bare-ended or conical tip fiber is used with 5 watts to 7 watts of power in the continuous mode. It is important to limit the laser exposure time to less than three seconds and to cool the fiber by immersion in sterile saline between exposures. Active fluid irrigation over the fiber tip site can also limit or elimi-

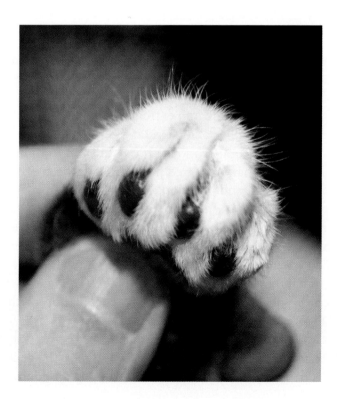

Figure 9-10 Diode laser-assisted onychectomy, 12 hours post-op.

nate excessive thermal injury and post-operative complications. The laser should not be activated unless the tip of the fiber is in direct contact with the tissue. This device can be successfully used for the procedure if these guidelines are followed.

Dissection and Removal of Internal and Subcutaneous Neoplasia

The diode laser is uniquely suited for the dissection and excision of subcutaneous and internal masses. The tactile control and feedback of this laser in the contact mode offers the ability to precisely approach and dissect these masses. Meticulous and precise hemostasis can be achieved. The effect of this laser is superior to that obtained with the carbon dioxide laser. Adequate hemostasis allows for better visualization of the surgical field and better identification of the abnormal tissue. Pancreatic, hepatic, and renal masses can be removed without excessive blood loss and with a reduced need for ligation and other hemostatic methods. Thyroidectomies and adrenalectomies are more easily performed with this laser. Hemostasis is more complete and surrounding tissues are not damaged. (Figure 9-11)

When a thyroidectomy is performed with a diode laser the blood supply to the adjacent parathyroid is easily preserved. This markedly reduces the risk of postoperative hypocalcemia. The surgical approach is performed in a routine manner.[22] The use of surgical loupes enhances the surgeon's ability to identify and preserve critical structures. The external parathyroid glands are identified and gently dissected free with the tip of the diode fiber. (Figure 9-11) The laser is activated only as required to provide hemostasis. A 600-micron, carbonized fiber with a setting of 2 to 3 watts is usually sufficient. The added advantage is the superior hemo-

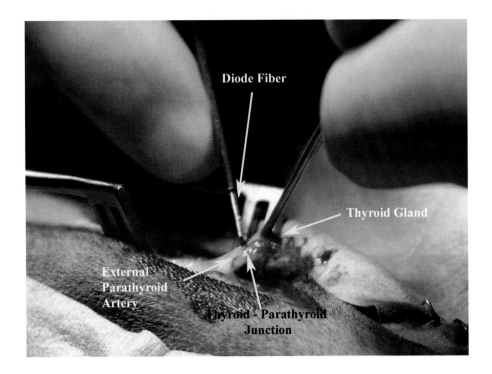

Figure 9-11 Diode laser-assisted thyroidectomy; dissection of the parathyroid gland preserving its vasculature.

stasis. Again, adequate cooling of the surgical area is imperative to avoid delayed tissue swelling or necrosis. After excision of the thyroid gland has been completed the internal parathyroid can be dissected free and transplanted into the cervical muscle. Care must be taken to only transplant the parathyroid gland without any thyroid tissue.

Generally speaking, neoplastic tissues are more highly vascularized than normal tissue. A tumor-free margin is required to completely excise the abnormal tissue. The size of the margin should be based on the suspected tumor type and the potential complications versus the benefits from the excision of normal tissue. The guidelines for the laser excision of neoplastic tissue to provide adequate clean margins should be no different from those used with conventional surgery.

A 600-micron fiber in the appropriate length handpiece is used in these procedures. The general guidelines for use are similar to those listed above. Power settings of between 3 watts and 14 watts are used, depending on the desired speed, precision, and vascularity of the target tissue. It should be noted that the rate at which the fiber can overheat is directly proportional to the power used and the exposure time. Higher powers and longer exposure can more rapidly overheat the fiber. Failure to adequately control the heat of the fiber will result in inadvertent peripheral thermal damage. Depending on the location, this can have catastrophic results in the post-operative period. Hemostasis is better obtained at lower powers (2 watts to 4 watts) with longer exposure times. Incision or excision is achieved at higher powers with shorter exposure times (6 watts to 14 watts with less than three seconds duration).

In cases where complete excision is not possible and the mass is highly pigmented or more vascular than the surrounding tissue, the diode laser can be used in a free-beam mode. In these cases a larger diameter fiber at higher powers is employed. Orb fibers are ideally suited for this procedure. This is somewhat dependent on the size of the tumor. In most cases a 600-micron or 1,000-micron fiber is used with power setting of 15 watts to 60 watts. The aiming beam should be used to precisely align the laser energy to the target. It is imperative to cool the fiber to prevent damage to the operator, the fiber, and the tissue. Any carbonization that forms on the surface of the tissue should be promptly removed between exposures. Absorption of the laser energy by the target tissue will cause vaporization of the surface tissues and coagulation and subsequent necrosis of the deeper tissue. This method is imprecise at best. Tissue as deep as 3 mm may be effected. It is imperative to consider the underlying structures and any related potential complications.

The diode laser can also be used to treat non-resectable solid tissue masses. This includes metastatic hepatic lesions. The coagulation status of the patient and the histopathologic diagnosis for the patient should be available prior to treatment. These lesions can be treated laparoscopically (see below) or during laparotomy. Fibers of 600 microns to 1,000 microns or special multi-fiber bundles can be used for this purpose. The fiber(s) are introduced into the lesion and sufficient laser energy is applied for a sufficient period of time to cause a blanched appearance in the target tissue. A good starting point is 12 watts for six seconds. In these cases the laser fiber will be cooled by thermal dilution in the tissue. This procedure is only palliative but when applied laprascopically has the potential to prolong the patient's life with minimal debilitation. Recent advances in monitoring the direct effect of laser energy on the tissue may expand the usefulness of this therapeutic modality in the future. Systems that monitor the temperature of the treated tissue and control the laser may prove useful.[23] Recently, a system has been developed to provide precise control and treatment planning using magnetic resonance imaging (MRI). Tissue temperatures are monitored and the laser is controlled by software that monitors MRI-calculated temperatures.[24,25]

Oral Surgery

Diode lasers can play an important role in oral surgery. As previously stated, the diode lasers most commonly used in veterinary surgery are preferentially absorbed by tissues containing hemoglobin, oxyhemoglobin, melanin, and to a much lesser extent, water. The oral mucosa contains abundant amounts of these substances.

Diode lasers can be used to remove oral masses (Figure 9-12), perform gingivectomies, create periodontal flaps, or treat periodontal disease. Generally, the laser is used in a contact mode to incise or excise tissue. The guidelines listed in the previous section apply. More efficient cutting is obtained by carbonization of the fiber tip. For incision and excision a 600-micron fiber in the appropriate handpiece is used. Power settings of 4 watts to 8 watts in the continuous wave mode are usually adequate for incision or excision. Specialized dental handpieces with a highly malleable tip are available. These handpieces allow for better access in smaller patients or tight locations. Standard surgical approaches and techniques should be observed. Use of the diode laser offers enhanced intra-operative hemostasis and improved post-operative patient comfort (Figure 9-13).

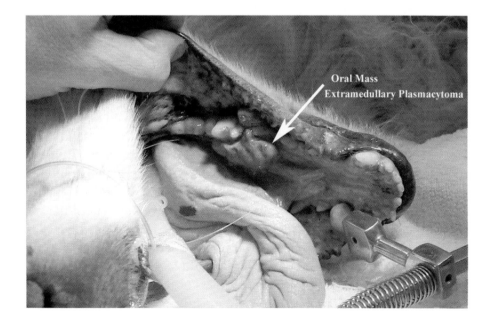

Figure 9-12 Oral mass, pre-treatment.

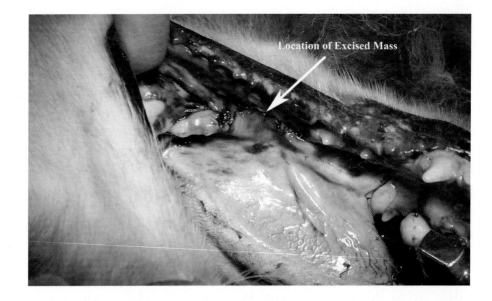

Figure 9-13 Appearance of surgical site post-operatively.

Lower power laser treatment has been shown to decrease the depth of the periodontal pocket, reduces inflammation, and appears to markedly decrease the amount of pathogenic bacteria.[26] I have no personal experience in treating periodontal pockets with the diode laser. This technique may prove safe and effective in the future.

Treatment of Canine and Feline Melanomas

The use of the diode laser in the treatment of oral melanoma in combination with immunotherapy may offer a unique opportunity for improved survival in this difficult and highly malignant process. The preferential absorption of diode laser energy by melanin allows the tumor cells to be specifically targeted. Standard oncological surgical guidelines should still be attempted in these cases.

Early and complete excision with evaluation of the draining lymph nodes still offers the best prognosis. A more rostral tumor location of smaller size and the absence of bone lysis have been shown to have increased survival times.[27] Complete resection with clean histologic margins, achieving local control with the first surgical attempt and no evidence of metastasis, offers the best long-term prognosis.[28] The diode lasers may enhance the opportunity to achieve local control with the first surgery (Figure 9-14). In the best scenario the tumor should be widely excised with the laser. Even in cases of wide excision it may be useful to expose the tumor bed to diode laser energy in a free-beam mode. In theory, any stray malignant melanin-containing cells would be preferentially destroyed by the laser energy. The areas are treated with a 1,000-micron fiber at 15 watts to 25 watts in the continuous wave mode until the surface of the tumor bed has a slightly blanched appearance. The fiber must be kept cool during this process by irrigation with saline and any carbonized tissue that forms on the surface should be removed between laser irradiation. Specially designed jacketed fibers or orb-tipped fibers are particularly useful in this application. Care must be taken not to overexpose

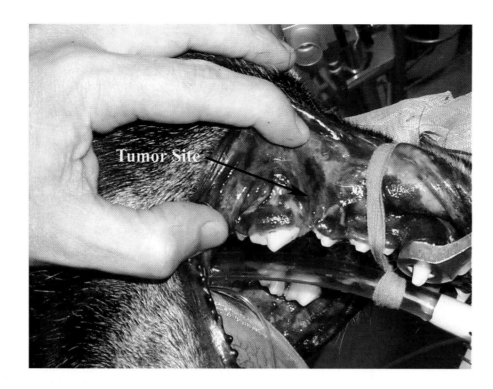

Tumor Site

Figure 9-14 Appearance of surgical site one month post-malignant melanoma removal.

these areas. Due to the depth of penetration into this application, the subsequent necrosis of devitalized tissues needs to be carefully considered.

In those cases where the melanoma has recurred locally and/or complete excision is not an option, this wavelength can offer palliation of clinical signs and may improve the patient's quality and duration of life. Treatment of these lesions can be accomplished by interstitial laser therapy (ILT) or in a free-beam mode. The choice of application depends on the depth, size, and location of the lesion. Excisional debridement followed by ILT or free-beam ablation, where possible, may offer the best chance for local control. In these cases follow-up radiation and/or chemotherapy should be considered. In the future, immunotherapy may offer substantially improved survival time for this disease.[29,30]

Oral malignant melanomas are rare in cats. These tumors should be approached in a similar fashion as their canine counterparts.[31] Complete excision on the first attempt with evaluation for metastasis to regional lymph nodes and pulmonary metastasis should be performed. Complete excision without evidence of metastasis probably offers the best prognosis.

Dermal melanomas can occur in both dogs and cats, but are rare. Digital melanomas have an increased risk of malignancy and may behave aggressively.[32] Because these tumors have a higher metastatic potential they should be treated aggressively with digital amputation and evaluation for metastasis to the draining lymph node and lungs. The diode laser can be used in the digital amputation. In both cases the technique is similar to the feline onychectomy. Immunotherapy may also improve survival in these cases. The combination of diode laser surgery and immunotherapy has led to the survival of one patient with malignant melanoma of the digit for more than five and one-half years. This patient had metastasis to the draining popliteal lymph node at the time of diagnosis. This response is particularly impressive when compared to the usual median survival time of twelve months.[33] As of this time, no investigations have been performed to evaluate the potential additional benefits of diode laser surgery over conventional techniques with or without the addition of immunotherapy.

Ophthalmologic Surgery

A complete discussion of the uses of the diode laser in ophthalmologic surgery is beyond the scope of this chapter. The reader is referred to general and specialty surgical texts for further information. Diode lasers have been used in the treatment of iris cysts, melanomas, and detached retinas (Figure 9-15). As an example, diode lasers can be used to control retinal bleeding without damaging corneal structures.

Minimally Invasive Surgical Techniques

Diode lasers are ideally suited for use in minimally invasive surgery. The fiber delivery system allows for the delivery of laser energy through various endoscopic and videoscopic devices. Many of these techniques are enhanced or occur in a fluid environment. As previously discussed, the preferential absorption by pigmented tissues allows for these systems to be used while immersed during irrigation. It is beyond the scope of this chapter to discuss the techniques and equipment involved in each minimally invasive procedure. Advanced training courses are available in these techniques. They should only be used by practitioners who have had adequate training and experience and have the proper endoscopic equipment. Diode lasers vastly expand the diagnostic and therapeutic abilities of minimally invasive surgery. Patient recovery time and discomfort are mini-

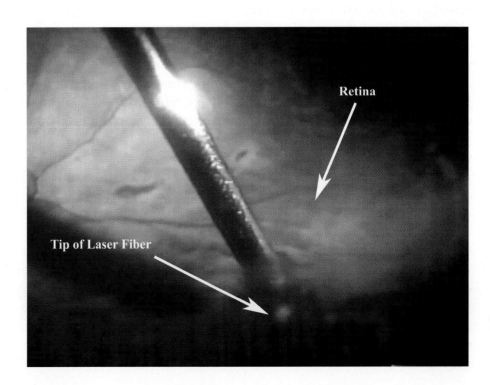

Figure 9-15 Retinal re-attachment (retinopexy) with the diode laser.

mized with these techniques. As the general public becomes increasingly aware of minimally invasive surgery, the demand for these services will increase.

The general principles of diode laser surgery as described in the previous sections still apply with any minimally invasive technique. It is imperative to control the heat generated by these fibers during lasing. The extraneous heat generated by these fibers during exposure may not only cause harm to the patient, but will result in damage to the endoscopic equipment. The amount of heat that the fiber generates is a function of the laser's power setting (power), the exposure time, the mode used (contact versus free-beam), and the target tissue or lasing environment (thermodilution). The heat generated by the fiber may be controlled in three ways: (1) by limiting the power utilized, (2) by controlling the exposure time, and (3) by cooling the fiber. Power should be sufficient to accomplish the procedure in a timely manner without causing inadvertent peripheral damage. Exposure times should be limited to less than approximately three seconds. The exact time depends on the other factors discussed (power, target tissue, and operating environment). Cooling of the fiber may be accomplished by either immersion with continuous irrigation or pulse irrigation of the fiber.

In addition, the laser should never be activated unless the tip of the fiber (active end) is outside of the operating channel of the endoscopic equipment. The fiber should be evaluated in a darkened room for any breaks along its length. The aiming beam should only be visible at the tip of the fiber. Visualization of the aiming beam anywhere along the length of the fiber indicates a fracture and laser energy will "leak" from these areas. Fractures along the length of the fiber will markedly reduce the amount of energy reaching the tip. The emanation of laser energy from these fractures may severely damage the endoscopic equipment and poses a hazard to operatory personnel. If the aiming beam is visualized anywhere along the length of the fiber, the fiber should be cleaved to this level or discarded.

Fiber selection depends on the procedure and may be limited based on the working channel of the endoscopic device. Fibers are readily available between 200 microns and 1,000 microns. A majority of these fibers are bare-ended. When used in the contact mode the tips of these fibers may be carbonized as previously described. Carbonization of the fiber tip enhances the thermal effect on non- or lightly pigmented tissue. Jacketed fibers are also available and are useful to provide adequate cooling for procedures requiring a free-beam, un-immersed mode.

Gastrointestinal Endoscopy

Pedunculated polyps within the colon can be resected with the diode laser. A 600-micron fiber with 3 watts to 6 watts of power in a continuous mode can generally be used. The fiber tip can be cooled with the endoscope's irrigation system. Any plume can be evacuated with endoscopic suction. By alternating irrigation and suction, the target tissue can be kept cool and any accumulated carbonization removed. The laser should only be activated when the tip of the fiber is fully extended and visible.

Activation of the laser with the fiber in the biopsy channel may result in severe damage to the endoscope. It is also important to perform this procedure carefully and avoid the perforation of the colon at the time of polypectomy. Caution must be taken to avoid excessive peripheral thermal damage to avoid colonic perforation at a later time. In most cases it is preferred to remove a majority of the mass with a snare or a biopsy instrument first and then remove the remaining abnormal tissue with the laser. This technique provides good hemostasis and decreases the risk of inadvertent perforation. Caution should be exercised depending on the depth of the abnormal tissue. Any excised tissue should be submitted for histopathologic evaluation.

Hemorrhaging ulcers within the stomach or gastrointestinal tract may also be controlled with the diode laser (Figure 9-16). A complete endoscopic evaluation within the gastrointestinal tract should be performed in these animals. Multiple biopsy specimens should be obtained from and directly adjacent to the ulcerated area. Additionally, biopsy samples should be taken for the stomach (cardia, fundus, pyloric antrum), small intestines, and colon. These samples should also be submitted for histopathology. The ulcerated area can be treated with a 1,000-micron fiber directly in contact with the bleeding area (3 watts to 8 watts) with one- to two-second exposure times. Continuous irrigation will help identify the vessel and control the heating of the fiber. In humans, these areas have also been treated in a free-beam mode with the laser fiber 0.5 to 1 cm from the target and 10 watts to 14 watts of power.[34] Excessive use of power or exposure times should be avoided to prevent inadvertent peripheral damage resulting in perforation. Care must be taken not to mechanically perforate the gastrointestinal tract with the laser fiber.

Laparoscopy

Diode lasers can be used laparoscopically to provide hemostasis, excise tissue, and for interstitial therapy (ILT) of non-resectable neoplasia. Hemo-

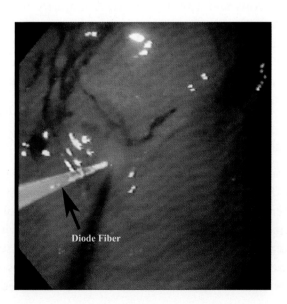

Figure 9-16 Endoscopic treatment of gastric ulcer.

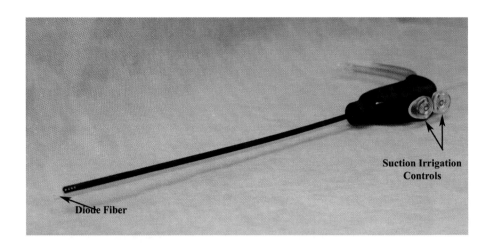

Figure 9-17 Laparoscopic suction, irrigation, and laser fiber guide.

stasis is critical to the success of any laparoscopic procedure; the diode laser provides for excellent hemostasis. The principles of use are the same as general surgery. Hemostasis is provided with lower power density for longer exposures. Excision is accomplished with higher power densities for shorter duration.

Generally fibers of 600 or 1,000 microns are used in this procedure. A 5 mm laparoscopic fiber guide is extremely useful in these cases (Figure 9-17). These fiber guides allow for precise placement of the fiber and can also be used to provide suction and irrigation of the operative site.[35] As with any procedure, cooling of the fiber and removal of carbonized tissue will help to minimize peripheral thermal damage. Control of fiber heating is accomplished, as previously discussed, by limiting exposure times and irrigating the fiber either during or between exposures.

Dissection of vascular structures (ovarian pedicles, testicular vasculature) can be accomplished by a combination of coagulation and excision. Blood vessels should be isolated by the appropriate use of blunt dissection. The isolated vessels are then coagulated in a contact or free-beam mode (Figure 9-18). The proximal aspect of the vessel is then grasped and the vessel is transected. The occlusion of the vessel is slowly released under direct observation. If any hemorrhaging is observed the vessel is re-grasped and additional laser energy is applied. If adequate hemostasis cannot be achieved an endoscopic ligaclip or ligature is placed. Larger vessels can be transected by placing two or three endoscopic ligaclips on the vessel and then transecting the vessel with the diode laser. This procedure provides an increased margin of safety for complete and adequate hemostasis.

The diode laser can provide excellent hemostasis after laparoscopic biopsy. The biopsy site can be treated in a contact or free-beam mode. In the contact mode a 600- or 1,000-micron bare-ended fiber in a 5 mm fiber guide is activated in contact with the hemorrhaging areas in the biopsy. The actively bleeding area is readily identified by the use of irrigation through the fiber guide. Three to six watts of laser energy are applied for three to six seconds. The fiber should be cooled during or between exposures by irrigation.

In the free-beam mode the fiber is aligned with the aiming beam and is

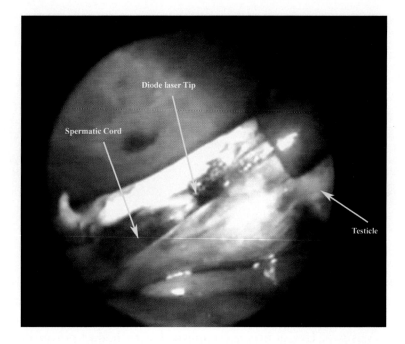

Figure 9-18 Laparoscopic transection of the spermatic cord of a cryptochid testicle with the diode laser.

positioned approximately 0.5 to 1 centimeter from the target. The fiber must be cooled by irrigation when used in this mode. Ten to fifteen watts of energy is applied until hemostasis is achieved. This will usually occur within three to five seconds. If the desired result does not occur in a reasonable time the contact mode or alternative methods of hemostasis should be considered.

Treatment of non-resectable hepatic malignances can be attempted with ILT. The beneficial effects of this treatment have not been well documented. It remains to be elucidated if patients treated in this manner have decreased morbidity, mortality, and longer median survival times than those receiving no treatment or chemotherapy. At this time this treatment should be regarded as experimental in animal patients and the client should be fully informed of the potential risks and benefits. In human patients ILT appears useful in the treatment of non-resectable hepatic metastases from colorectal cancer and hepatocellular carcinoma. It appears to improve survival times and is potentially less debilitating.[36,37,38] Recent advances in real-time temperature monitoring and control with magnetic resonance imaging may enhance the usefulness of this modality in the future.[39,40] The treatment of human benign prostatic hypertrophy with a diode-laser-coupled computer-controlled temperature-sensing fiber has been shown to be useful in the treatment of these lesions.[41] This technique and equipment might also prove useful in the treatment of non-resectable lesions in companion animals.

In these cases a laser fiber is introduced into the approximate center of the mass and 10 to 15 watts of laser energy is used. Exposure times vary with the size of the mass. In MRI-regulated studies on experimentally induced brain tumors in dogs, a laser "conditioning" prior to the main exposure appeared to allow for higher treatment powers to be used for ILT. The exposure used to pre-treat was 0.5 watts for one minute.[42] This appeared to be clinically useful in these cases. Well controlled studies and comparisons of pretreated versus non-pretreated tissues are not available. The end point for treatment is the observation that normal tissue directly adjacent to the mass just begins to lighten in color. The variability seen in power and exposure times may be due to the size of the lesion and the degree of perfusion of the tissue. These treatments might also prove useful in the palliative treatment of canine prostatic malignancies and other non-resectable masses that are non-responsive to other treatment modalities. ILT appears to have a low complication rate and good post-operative patient comfort. Whether or not this treatment increases median life expectancy in these cases remains to be seen.

Rigid Endoscopy (Otoendoscopy, Rhinoscopy, Cystoscopy, Arthroscopy)

The diode laser is especially useful in these procedures. It can treat disease processes that would otherwise require more extensive, invasive, and debilitating surgeries. These procedures are usually carried out in a fluid environment, which makes the diode laser ideal. As previously noted, irrigation provides for optimal fiber cooling, which allows higher laser energies to be applied to the target tissue, for the result is more rapid and complete treatment while still maintaining the advantages of laser surgery. Under continuous or intermittent irrigation, sources of hemorrhage are rapidly identifiable and usually easily coagulated. Immersion in a fluid environment also increases visualization of the treatment area. In this environment tissue is removed as it is lased, and any carbonized tissue can be rapidly removed, helping to minimize peripheral thermal damage. Diode lasers can be used in rigid endoscopy to incise or ablate tissue. They also provide for excellent hemostasis. (Figures 9-19 and 9-20)

In almost all cases the laser energy is provided in a contact mode. Fibers of any size can be used depending on the size of the lesion and the operating channel in the endoscope. The surgeon is again cautioned to be familiar with and adequately trained in these techniques and the use of the laser prior to attempting to perform any procedure. It is imperative to be

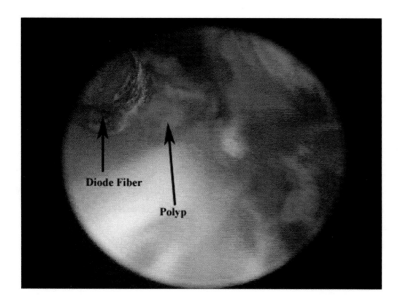

Figure 9-19 Diode ablation of a feline hyperplastic nasal polyp during video rhinoscopy.

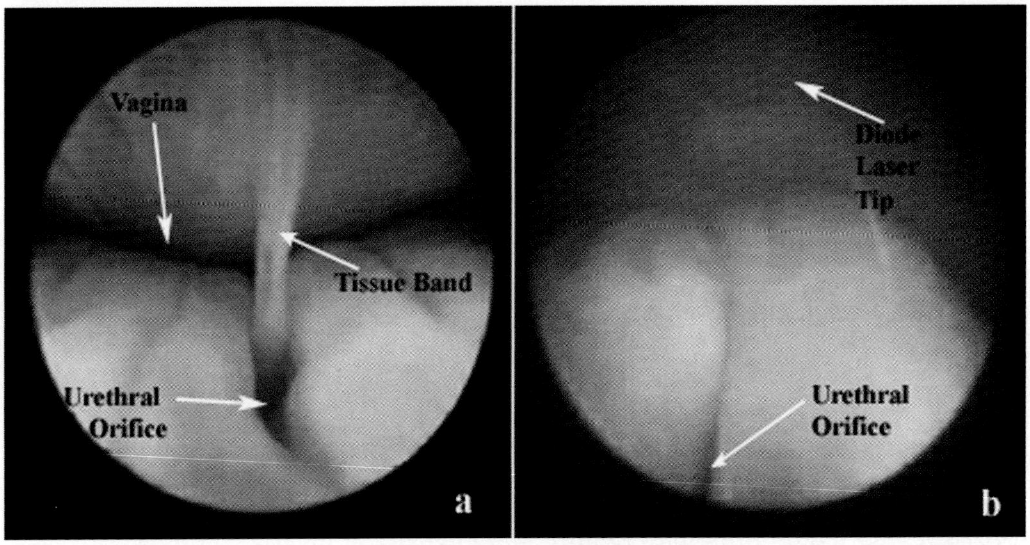

Figure 9-20 Urethral adhesion with fibrous tissue band pre- (a) and during (b) diode laser treatment.

able to visualize the tip of the fiber during the application of laser energy. Failure to do so may result in inadvertent peripheral damage to the endoscopic equipment.

Hemostasis can be rapidly accomplished with powers of 3 watts to 6 watts in a contact mode. Sufficient irrigation should be provided to allow for visualization of the source of the bleeding and prevent overheating of the fiber. Bubbles should never be seen forming at the tip of the fiber. If present, these indicate that the irrigant has been heated to the boiling point. If adequate irrigation is provided, exposure time is less critical. Hemostasis is usually achieved within three seconds if the tip of the fiber is properly positioned. The usefulness of the hemostatic effect of the diode lasers in these procedures cannot be overstated. Visualization of abnormal structures and their complete removal is greatly enhanced with this therapeutic modality.

Laser excision of masses can be accomplished in two ways. The mass can be removed with a biopsy instrument and the tumor bed then treated with the laser. This controls any hemorrhaging and should remove any abnormal tissue that remains. With this method post-operative patient comfort seems to be equivalent to direct excision. Polypoid masses can sometimes also be directly excised at their bases with the diode laser. Biopsy specimens should be obtained prior to any laser treatment, and submitted for histopathology.

Masses that have been proven to be benign can be removed by laser ablation or ILT. This involves introducing the fiber into the middle of the mass and firing the diode laser at 10 watts to 25 watts until the tissue has a blanched appearance. The devitalized tissue can then be removed with biopsy forceps and the site evaluated for complete excision. After debridement, hemostasis can be achieved as described above.

In combination with video otoscopy, diode lasers increase the surgeon's ability to treat auricular disease. The ability to resect abnormal tissue is greatly enhanced. Large auricular masses and hypertrophied tissue can be successfully resected with little or no debilitation to the patient (Figures

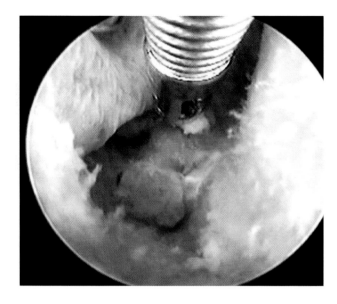

Figure 9-21 Canine ear polyp.

9-21 and 9-22). In addition, narrowing of the auricular canal can be corrected, allowing for the reduction in future occurrences of otitis externa. It is imperative to treat any underlying allergy or infection problems that may contribute to the patient's condition. A complete text on the use of lasers and video otoscopy is available and the practitioner is referred to this resource for further information.[43]

In addition to the ear canal, masses that arise from the middle ear can be readily treated if a small enough video otoscope is available. In general, a 2.7 mm, 30 degree rigid pediatric cystoscope (Figure 9-23) with an eleven french operating sheath provides for excellent access to the middle ear. This device allows for simultaneous irrigation and suction during these procedures. In my hands the diode laser is superior to the CO_2 in the treatment of ear diseases within the auricular canal and the osseous bulla (Figure 9-24).

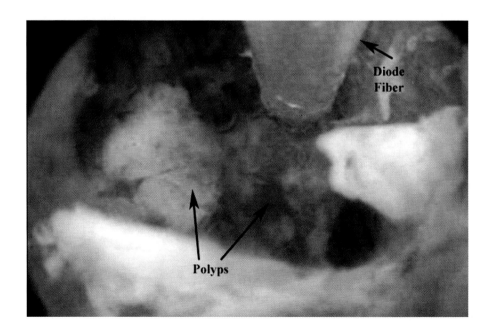

Figure 9-22 Ear polyp removal with diode laser.

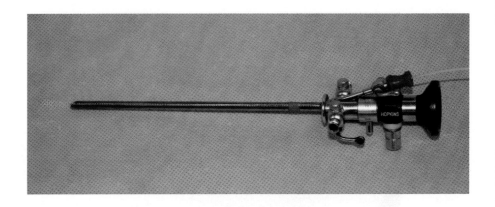

Figure 9-23 Pediatric cystoscope with operating channel.

ILT can also prove useful in the palliative treatment of malignant neoplastic processes, such as nasal osteosarcoma or nasal or aural adenocarcinoma. This should be reserved for non-resectable neoplasia or cases in which the pet owner has elected not to proceed with standard (laser) oncologic surgical procedures. In these cases, tumor mass can be temporarily reduced with little or no debilitation to the patient. The procedure is performed as indicated above. In one case of nasal osteosarcoma the patient survived for eighteen months and maintained an excellent quality of life, jogging with the owner on an almost daily basis. This spayed female golden retriever was 20 months old at the time of definitive diagnosis. She had two rhinoscopic procedures for laser tumor debridement and ILT. (Figure 9-25) The median survival time of dogs with axial osteosarcoma treated with surgery alone was twenty-two weeks.[44] The median survival time in dogs treated with palliative radiation was 162 days.[45] In another, smaller study, large breed dogs treated with definitive radiation therapy had a median survival of 265 days.[46] The results of this one case far exceed those seen in these studies. Further study is warranted to determine if this outcome is reproducible in a larger patient sample. If this one result is representative, then laser treatment could offer a viable alternative to current modalities. Post-operative comfort was excellent and no untoward side effects were noted.

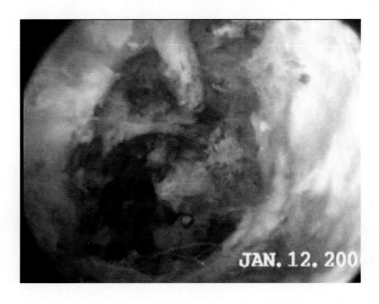

Figure 9-24 Middle ear after diode mass removal.

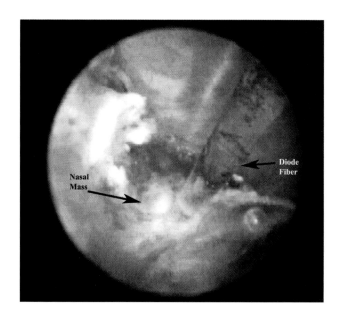

Figure 9-25 ILT with diode laser for nasal tumor.

Photodynamic Therapy

Photodynamic therapy (PDT) is defined as "a form of cancer treatment using a photosensitizing agent administered intravenously which concentrates selectively in tumor cells, followed by exposure of the tumor tissue to a special red laser light, in order to destroy as much of the tumor as possible."[47] This form of therapy allows for the selective targeting of abnormal tissue. The photosensitizing agent is injected intravenously into the patient. The agent is then activated by exposure to the appropriate wavelength of laser light. This produces a photochemical reaction that causes cell death.

PDT has been used in veterinary and human oncology to treat a large variety of neoplastic processes including prostatic carcinoma,[48] canine transitional cell carcinoma,[49] intranasal tumors,[50] and skin tumors.[51] This therapy is still in the investigational stages, but early results have been promising. It may offer the ability to uniquely target and destroy abnormal tissue. The usefulness of this treatment will depend on the development and identification of selective photosensitizers and the availability of cost-effective diode lasers.

Notes

1. The Diode Laser—The First Thirty Days Forty Years Ago. Dupuis, Russell D., IEEE Leos Newsletter, Vol 17 Number 1, Feb. 2003 Piscataway, NJ. http://www.ieee.org/organizations/pubs/newsletters/leos/feb03/diode.html

2. CORD Laser/Electro-Optics Technology Series. Cord Communications, 324 Kelly Drive, P.O. Box 21206, Waco, Texas 76702-1206. http://repairfaq.ece.drexel.edu/sam/CORD/leot/course03_mod11/mod03-11.html

3. Transendoscopic laser ablation of upper respiratory cysts in 12 horses, 1993-2003. Tate Jr, Lloyd P., Proc. SPIE Vol. 5312, p. 354-358.

4. Endometrial Cysts in the Mare. Stanton, Mary Beth, DVM; John V. Steiner, DVM, Dipl ACT; D.G. Pugh, DVM, MS, Dipl ACT, ACVN; J Equine Vet Sci 24[1]:14-19 Jan 2004.

5. Large Animal and Emerging Applications for Lasers. Bartels, Kenneth E., Western Veterinary Conference 2002.

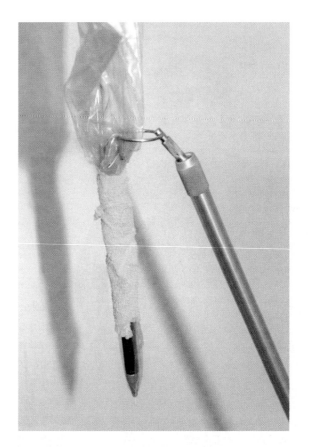

Figure 10-3 Straight hand piece attached to hollow waveguide and readied for aseptic use.

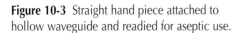

inate some char. Tips can be cold sterilized between uses in an appropriate disinfectant solution, but must be completely dry before use. The increasing supply of tips has lowered their cost, so it is wise to discard the tip after a few uses and incorporate that cost into the operating expense of the laser. It is contraindicated to use faulty tips that will cause excessive heating of target tissues or damage to the hollow flexible waveguide. Finally, for the purpose of convenience, it is practical to keep a tackle box nearby to neatly organize the tips and other accessories in one compact area.

A sterile surgical pack including an additional handpiece, instruments, gauze, and sterile saline should always be available at the beginning of every laser surgery procedure (Figure 10-4).

It is essential to have this ready to wipe away any char that forms at the edges of the incision. Because char is a tissue irritant, leaving it within incisions may lead to wound dehiscence. Moistened gauze also is used as a barrier to absorb any stray beams of laser energy during a procedure. This serves to protect nearby structures from inadvertent thermal injury.

It is also important to use an octylated cyanoacrylate following CO_2 laser surgery. It is most useful in feline declaw procedures and routine spay and neuter procedures. Octylated cyanoacrylate is a clear tissue adhesive which functions differently than the regular blue, butylated cyanoacrylate. Because a laser incision that is made correctly will be clean and dry, this clear, uncolored skin closure product allows the incision edges to remain in opposition. It will not be effective if the wound edges are oozing or bloody. Also, it is not to be buried under the skin; therefore, when used in the feline declaw procedure it must only be applied to the dry and clean incision edges. If the incision is not made correctly, or if there is remaining char at the wound edges, there will be surgical complications, e.g., wound dehiscence.

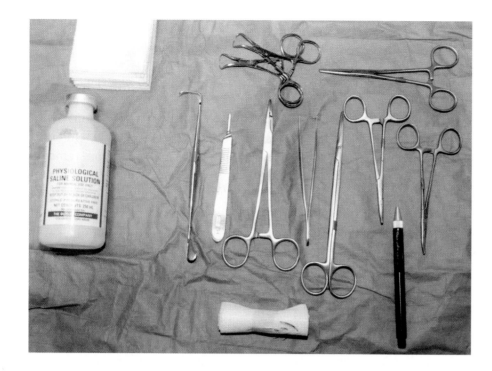

Figure 10-4 Standard surgical pack preparation for use with CO_2 laser energy.

In general, any incision is enhanced with the superpulse (SP) temporal pattern, available with an appropriately equipped CO_2 laser unit. Because the superpulse temporal pattern creates sharp and rapid peaks of intensity followed by intermittent rests, there is an optimal balance of vaporization and thermal relaxation of target tissues. To create an incision with the laser the surgeon should produce tension at the leading edge of the beam that vaporizes tissues. This causes the characteristic clean and dry charred separation of tissue at the zone of vaporization. The zones of thermal necrosis and thermal conduction are thus greatly diminished and create a superior incision with negligible thermal effects to surrounding tissues. There is some superficial char formation when superpulse mode is used; however, it is almost completely removed by gentle wiping of wound edges with sterile moistened gauze. Some surgeons may also prefer to repeat the superpulse mode (30 Hz, 25 msec pulse width = 75% power) to add more control when making an incision in a delicate anatomical area (e.g., for stenotic nare correction or ferret adrenalectomy).

In contrast, when continuous wave (CW) or repeated pulse temporal patterns (PW) are used, there is greater carbonization of tissues and more char remains. These settings also cause slightly larger zones of thermal necrosis and thermal conduction for an equivalent zone of vaporization. Therefore, a higher degree of incisional hemostasis should be expected compared to an incision made using superpulse mode. If superpulse is not available, the surgeon may still wish to minimize char formation created with incisions. Several repeat pulse settings are available on all CO_2 laser units. After experimenting with several settings, we have found that 40% power repeat pulse (20 Hz, 20 msec pulse width) is the closest setting to superpulse available at this time. A table of common settings is available in the user's manual supplied by the manufacturer.

There are many surgical procedures not described herein that are performed better with a surgical CO_2 laser. We are continually impressed with the efficiency of this surgical laser wavelength. Many areas of the body that are generally perceived as difficult by other means due to bleeding tendencies are now manageable; the eye, ear, nose, and throat are the most commonly cited. Skin fold-plasty, incisions for lipoma removal, and treatment of furunculosis are all common cosmetic procedures easily performed with a laser. Besides skin incision for surgical sterilization, my favorite laser surgical procedures are cystotomy, thyroidectomy, elongated soft palate correction, anal sacculectomy, perianal adenoma removal, acral lick granuloma, and indolent ulcer treatment, because there is minimal or no hemorrhage during the procedure and visibility is unsurpassed. The potential for important future innovative procedures is enormous.

We have observed that by using a CO_2 laser the patient's post-surgical comfort is dramatically improved over traditional techniques. More detailed studies are needed to organize and document these findings. A new discipline of veterinary surgery is unfolding before us. At no other time in history have pets been anthropomorphized as the present. It is every veterinarian's responsibility to minimize animal suffering in any way possible. Therefore, if CO_2 laser surgery is truly a superior technique in its appropriate application, it should be used as an everyday tool for surgical procedures such as skin tumor removal, sexual sterilization, and feline declaw.

Surgical Technique

Having a good understanding of the physical properties associated with laser-tissue interaction is a must to achieve the most favorable surgical outcome possible. Once this has been accomplished the clinician can then undertake the relatively short learning curve (two to four weeks) needed to become technically proficient with a surgical laser.

Each laser has specific requirements for the appropriate distance between the handpiece and target tissue. Consult the manufacturers specifications for optimal focal point parameters. As previously discussed, the position of the laser handpiece should be maintained in as perpendicular a fashion as possible to maximize correct beam geometry. Severe angulation of the laser beam will not only stress the armature, but also create a focal distance disparity between the leading and trailing edges of the laser beam. This could greatly impact the lasers' vaporization potential to the target tissue. An uneven power density distribution will result and potentially create a leading edge of desiccation and contracture of tissue. Remember that distance, power, and appeture diameter of the handpiece all play a critical interactive role in power density.

A great advantage of laser energy is the ability of the clinician to minimize excessive tissue manipulation. For initial incisions, undermining tissue and adequate tissue tension at a 45° to 90° angle will optimize tissue vaporization by improving tissue separation upon vaporization. An additional benefit is a general reduction in char formation. Too much tension could result in tissue tearing, rupturing small vessels and tearing nociceptors and lymphatic vessels. This can effectively negate the promoted positive laser tissue effects previously outlined.

Clinicians new to laser tissue interaction should become accomplished at routine skin incisions, muscle and fat dissection, and tissue undermining before attempting more complex uses of laser-tissue interaction. Having a comfortable working knowledge of distance manipulation to change from vaporization to collagen contracture, protein denaturation, and coagulation before attempting surgery in highly vascular or recessed areas will bode well for a positive surgical outcome.

As the laser energy vaporizes tissue, peripheral tissue-energy interaction provides nocieceptor sealing, vessel contracture, and small lymphatic vessel sealing. All these promote positive tissue handling interaction. Conversely, excessive peripheral thermal tissue effect will delay or create failure of proper wound healing, in some cases severely increasing potentials for incisional dehiscence.

Some success can be achieved with nonspecific granulation tissue bleeding by applying laser energy in the 500 to 1,500 power density range. Again, learning to paint a vascular area with adequate laser energy to seal small bleeding vessels can improve time management of a multitude of surgical cases.

Standard protocols for use of CO_2 laser energy in small animal clinical practice has been validated by numerous individuals, all using similar spot diameters, power settings, and power output modes to achieve positive therapeutic outcomes. A currently accepted technique chart is provided.

Routine Procedure Considerations

Today's demanding pet owner desires the finest care available in medical technology and surgery. The recent availability of more affordable, compact CO_2 surgical laser technology has provided practitioners with a new and exciting way to satisfy their clients' desire for high-quality medicine. Today's veterinary CO_2 laser equipment is relatively easy to master as a surgical tool, and its post-operative benefits engender a lasting impression of compassionate care in the pet-owner's mind.

Here we introduce some suggested techniques for elective surgical procedures that all veterinary practitioners can perform every day using a CO_2 laser. In general, the techniques vary little from standard protocol, with the exception that a scalpel-like handpiece delivering focused laser energy replaces the traditional steel scalpel.

Table 10-1 General parameters for CO_2 laser use

Routine incision:	Routine ablation/vaporization
Spot Diameter: 0.4 mm	Spot Diameter: 0.8 mm
Power Setting: 6 to 10 W	Power Setting: 10 to 20 W
Power Output: Continuous wave	Power Output: Continuous wave
+/_ superpulse	(Use pulsed wave in delicate areas)
Delicate location incision:	**Routine excision:**
Spot Diameter: 0.3 to 0.4 mm	Spot Diameter: 0.8 mm
Power Setting: 3 to 6 W	Power Setting: 8 to 15 W
Power Output: Pulse wave	Power Output: Continuous wave
Superpulse	(non-superpulse enhances hemostasis)

We use a 20 W CO_2 laser with superpulse capability. This produces an intense, monochromatic, coherent, collimated beam of infrared light at a wavelength of 10.6 μm. The laser beam is delivered to the surgical site via a hollow flexible waveguide that terminates at a scalpel-like handpiece. The laser energy exits the handpiece through exchangeable tube-shaped tips (various diameters ranging from 0.3 mm to 1.4 mm). The various suggested focusing tip sizes will be indicated so that proper power density can be delivered. The power settings that are given here are suggested guidelines for use and **not** absolute values for the given procedure.

The mode of energy delivery is described as either CW (continuous wave), meaning that the laser is delivering a continuous stream of laser power, or as CW SP (continuous wave, superpulse), a stream of laser energy characterized by a pattern of sharp and rapid peaks and rests of laser energy intensity. Superpulse provides an optimal balance of vaporization (peaks) and thermal relaxation (rests) of target tissues, thereby minimizing tissue charring and collateral thermal necrosis. If superpulse is not available, then a continuous wave, pulsed wave (CW PW) can be delivered, which also provides for a period of rest and cooling between pulses, but is not as effective in reducing heat and char formation. See Chapter 4 for more detailed explanations of thermal accumulation and thermal relaxation.

The CO_2 laser wavelength has a high absorption coefficient in water that makes it ideal for soft tissue incisions and ablations because it results in the least amount of collateral tissue damage and post-operative coagulative necrosis due to heat. Because this particular wavelength does not pass through cellular water but strongly reacts with it, it vaporizes tissue layer-by-layer, minimizing energy transmission to underlying cellular structures.

On the other hand, wavelengths generated by diode or Nd:YAG (between 810 nm and 1,064 nm) lasers are poorly absorbed by cellular water, and react more with the pigments present in tissues. Due to the fact that cells are comprised more of water than pigments, these wavelengths more readily transmit through and scatter deeper within the tissue. Coagulative necrosis and deeper, more prolonged thermal conduction characterize the effects to tissue following irradiation at these wavelengths. The ability to deliver these wavelengths via optical quartz fiber makes them well suited to flexible endoscopic applications, and their high absorption in pigmented tissue makes them more efficient coagulators of larger blood vessels. However, the CO_2 laser's more predictable, controllable soft tissue effect, coagulative properties, broader range of applications, and inherently shorter learning curve make it the ideal laser for the general veterinary practitioner, and is the reason we prefer it over other wavelengths.

As discussed before, an understanding of standard skin incisions, excisions, and tissue undermining gives new users great confidence to expand their surgical use of lasers.

CO_2 laser use on the integumentary system is one of the most common uses in general clinical veterinary practice. Skin has 87% to 92% water component and thus is an exceptional target tissue for CO_2 laser energy.

Skin incisions should, whenever possible, be made with a spot diameter of less than 0.8 mm under slight tension. Adequate power density will allow a smooth single pass full thickness dermal penetration with minimal char. The non-contact aspect of CO$_2$ laser energy also reduces tissue distortion, especially in delicate regions on the body surface. We prefer to use a 0.4 mm spot size with superpulse continuous wave parameters when producing a skin incision.

Excisional parameters use the skin incision technique just described along with undermining of subcutaneous fat and connective tissue using a 0.8 mm spot size at adequate power density to continue adequate vaporization. Superpulse continuous wave mode is turned off at this point to improve hemostasis and enhance coagulation of small blood vessels. Continuing to provide light tension at a 45° to 90° angle with brown Addison forceps will allow for clean, efficient vaporization and removal of the tissue to be excised.

Tissue undermining provides for improved dermal release for wound closure. The CO$_2$ can provide excellent vaporization of connective tissue deep to the dermis. A 0.4 mm to 0.8 mm spot size is optimal for this technique. The laser beam should be parallel to the dermis and at the level of the connective tissue interface. Adequate tissue tension on the skin in an upward lifting motion will allow adequate visualization and access for vaporization. Be sure not to travel the laser beam too close to the dermis because peripheral thermal energy release may damage dermal blood supply.

Specific Surgical Case Management

Urogenital

Ovariohysterectomy

A routine spay in any patient is improved by using a laser because it reduces the post-operative pain, bleeding, and swelling. Make a midline skin incision using 0.4 mm tip, 6 W to 8 W CW SP. The surgeon may wish to use 7 W to 9 W SP pulsed 30Hz, 25 msec pulse width (75% power) to further reduce char formation, thermal conduction through tissue, and creation of laser surgical plume. After wiping away any char, the subcutaneous tissues are dissected away to clearly expose the linea alba. The abdominal muscles and peritoneum are tented up with forceps and a single cranial stab incision is created with a scalpel blade. Alternately, the handpiece can be angled to be close to parallel with the linea leading up to the tented region. Then a brief burst of 7 W to 9 W CW SP CO$_2$ laser energy is provided into the linea. This creates a laser stab incision. A grooved director is introduced into the abdominal incision to serve as a backstop for the CO$_2$ laser-assisted continuation of the incision. All internal structures must be protected from stray laser beams. Inadvertent lasing of the spleen, bladder, or mesenteric blood vessels could prove disastrous and should be avoided. The abdomen is incised using 0.4 mm tip 6 W to 8 W CW over the backstop, which is lifted upward to tense the targeted muscles and linea that are vaporized. Any char is wiped away from the clean and dry muscle edges. The procedure is then routinely continued. A surgeon may wish to vaporize tissues of the ovarian pedicle and/or cervical stump following ligation, although it is not recommended due to the larger diameter of the target vessels. Using the CO_2 laser to bisect the broad ligament can greatly reduce seepage from small blood vessels in the broad ligament. Pain receptors can also be sealed, reducing post-operative discomfort.

Following routine closure of the abdominal muscles and subcutis using absorbable suture material, the skin can be opposed with sutures; however, no exterior sutures may be necessary if tissue adhesive is used as a protective bandage. This technique has two benefits: it gives the client an added convenience because there is no need for a second visit to remove sutures, and the appearance of the surgical site is more pleasing. Because there is no swelling of the incision edges, incisions made with a surgical laser oppose cosmetically. (See Case Studies 12, 24.)

Feline Castration

After the patient is anesthetized and the scrotum is surgically prepped a single pass is made on the scrotal median raphe' using a 0.3 mm tip and 3 W to 4 W CW SP, or a 0.4 mm tip and 6 W to 8 W CW SP. Both testicles can be manually extracted, one at a time, through the same scrotal incision. Two separate incisions may be required in the scrotal subcutaneous tissues to completely exteriorize each testicle and supporting structures. Tension is applied to the testicular vessels by gentle traction of the testicle. Sterile moistened gauze is placed under the tensed scrotal cord to protect the surgeon. A single pass is made through the tunic to divide the testicular artery and vein as well as the vas deferens and cremaster muscle. The proximal remnant of the transected structures will retract through the inguinal ring into the abdomen. The vessels and nerves will be sealed immediately, causing hemostasis and diminished or absent pain.

Occasionally, a mature cat that has well-developed gonadal tissue and broad vasculature will bleed from the vaporizing pass made with a laser if the surgeon does not consider the diameter of the vessel. This occurs because the CO_2 laser seals only vessels that are smaller than the diameter of the laser tip being used for the incision. To vaporize the spermatic cord the surgeon may wish to use a 0.8 mm tip; use a ligature to be safest.

Any char remaining on the skin incision is wiped away with sterile moistened gauze. The edges are left in opposition and neither sutures nor surgical adhesive is required. The predominant benefit of using a laser in this technique is patient comfort and diminished bleeding. The surgeon should choose the technique carefully in a mature cat, and consider ligating the testicular vessels if they are large. Either way, if the scrotal incision is made using a laser, the patient will be more comfortable following the procedure. (See Case Study 6.)

Canine Anterior Scrotal Open Castration

A routine neuter in any patient is improved using a CO_2 laser because it diminishes the usual post-operative pain, bleeding, and swelling. The fur surrounding the entire scrotum is clipped and prepped atraumatically. We have found that most irritation to the scrotum is associated with excessive scrubbing and harsh chemicals. A 0.9% NaCl wash is applied to clean off any remaining soap or alcohol. Excessive or close clipping will initiate a cycle of irritation and self-mutilation in the patient, and should be avoided. The scrotum and surrounding exposed area is surgically prepped with a chlorhexidine scrub solution. One testicle is advanced to the anterior scrotal median raphe and used to create tension on the thinned scrotum where the incision is planned. A midline anterior scrotal incision is created with a 0.4mm tip using 6 W to 8 W CW SP. As the testicle tenses the scrotal skin, the incision is continued until the testicle begins to exteriorize. This should be accomplished in a single pass incision. The testicle is manually extracted through an incision in the scrotal subcutaneous tissue. The entire testicle and contents of the tunic are exteriorized and the connective tissue and any fat is wiped out and away with sterile gauze. The vaginal tunic is opened to clearly visualize the pampiniform plexus, vas deferens, and cremaster muscle. The cremaster muscle is ligated proximally with absorbable suture material and transected; or in dogs with light musculature, the cremaster can be cleanly divided using the laser beam. The pampiniform plexus and vas deferens are ligated and transected proximally as well.

The open castration of the second testicle is then performed through the same scrotal incision. A second incision is made in the scrotal subcutaneous tissue using the same surgical laser settings. The second testicle, likewise, is then surgically removed by open technique. Before final closure, the scrotum is examined for any bleeding or remaining fatty connective tissue. Any char is wiped from the incision edges. A small bead of tissue adhesive is placed over the incision to complete the procedure.

When performing laser-assisted castration on a mature dog, an experienced laser surgeon may consider using the same technique as in the young dog. Alternately, a preputial incision to advance the testicles through can be used, but this requires placement of a non-irritating subcutaneous absorbable suture to keep the incision edges opposed during healing. Proper use of the laser produces a clean and dry incision that heals rapidly. However, some dogs insist on grooming, which must be prevented to allow normal healing. An Elizabethan collar may be worn to prevent self-mutilation. (See Case Study 5.)

Canine Posterior Scrotal Open Castration

In an attempt to minimize patient-induced tissue irritation to a scrotal laser approach, we have found that this type of approach through the scrotal tissue allows for less access for the patient, while allowing easier visualization of the surgical incision by the owner. The fur surrounding the entire scrotum is clipped and prepped atraumatically. We have found that most irritation to the scrotum is associated with excessive scrubbing and harsh chemicals. A 0.9% NaCl wash is applied to clean off any remaining soap or alcohol. Excessive or close clipping will initiate a cycle of irritation and self-mutilation in the patient, and should be avoided. The scrotum and surrounding exposed area is surgically prepped with a chlorhexidine scrub solution. One testicle is advanced to the posterior scrotal median raphe adjacent to the surrounding integument and used to create tension on the thinned scrotum where the incision is planned. A midline posterior scrotal incision is created with a 0.4 mm tip using 6 W to 8 W CW SP. As the testicle tenses the scrotal skin, the incision is continued until the testicle begins to exteriorize. The total length of the incision can be as small as 1 centimeter due to the elasticity of the scrotal tissue. This should be accomplished in a single pass incision. The testicle is manually extracted through an incision in the scrotal subcutaneous tissue. The entire testicle and contents of the tunic are exteriorized and the connective tissue and any fat are wiped out and away with sterile gauze. The vaginal tunic is opened to clearly visualize the pampiniform plexus, vas deferens, and cremaster muscle. The cremaster muscle is ligated proximally with absorbable suture material and transected; or in dogs with light musculature the cremaster can be cleanly divided using the laser beam. Our personal experience indicates that the use of the CO2 laser beam without any crushing or ligation of the tissue allows for less postoperative pain. The pampiniform plexus and vas deferens are ligated and transected proximally as well.

The open castration of the second testicle is then performed through the same scrotal incision. A second incision is made in the scrotal subcutaneous tissue, through the original scrotal skin incision, using the same surgical laser settings. The second testicle, likewise, is then surgically removed by open technique. Before final closure, the scrotum is examined for any bleeding or remaining fatty connective tissue. Any char is wiped from the incision edges. A small bead of tissue adhesive is placed over the incision to complete the procedure.

When performing laser-assisted castration on a mature dog, use the same technique as in a young dog neuter. An experienced laser surgeon may consider continuing to use the scrotal approach. If the surgeon is uncomfortable with this incision style in a mature dog, a preputial incision to advance the testicles through can be used. This will require placement of a non-irritating subcutaneous absorbable suture to keep the incision edges opposed during healing. Proper use of the laser produces a clean and dry incision that heals rapidly. However, some dogs insist on grooming, which must be prevented to allow normal healing. An Elizabethan collar may be worn to prevent self-mutilation. (Review Case Study 5 with modifications listed above.)

Cystotomy

Perhaps the single most overlooked surgical procedure that is spectacularly enhanced with CO_2 laser is the cystotomy. Typically patients have a long history of hematuria during the diagnostic phase of care. By the time the patient has been selected as a surgical candidate for cystotomy the urinary bladder muscles are thickened from chronic muscle spasm, fibrosis, and edema. The mucosa is also frequently infected. Typical diseases of the bladder that require a corrective cystotomy include cystic calculi, polypoid cystitis, apical diverticulum, transitional cell carcinoma, and ectopic ureter(s). The classic post-surgical cystotomy patient continues to have significant hematuria for a few days. This is eliminated when the CO_2 laser is used. Because the laser incision is clean and dry there is no source of bleeding into the bladder following cystotomy. There is also reduced inflammation and contamination because the laser seals lymphatics and blood vessels and sterilizes the incision edges as it cuts. Because nerve endings are also sealed following laser incision, there is significantly less postoperative discomfort. The procedure is certainly more efficient because the laser surgeon does not spend time blotting out capillary bleeding. Visibility is enhanced because the clean and dry wound edges are not distorted. Pet owners are extremely satisfied following a curative procedure, and because chronic hematuria is seemingly resolved instantly following indicated laser cystotomy, this technique should be enthusiastically promoted when surgery is required.

The surgical approach to the bladder is slightly different for male dogs and female dogs. A routine caudal midline laparotomy is performed in the female dog. In the male dog, however, the prepuce covers the surgical exposure to the caudal midline. The caudal hypogastric vein also courses below the skin adjacent to the prepuce, and can cause bleeding during a procedure or bruising following a procedure because it has been ligated. Once again, the CO_2 laser provides a unique solution to this problem. The midline incision is created with a 0.4 mm spot size, 6 W to 8 W, CW SP, and courses sigmoidally to avoid the prepuce. Once the caudal hypogastric vein is identified it is ablated along with subcutaneous fat with a 0.8 mm spot size, 6 W to 8 W CW. The incision is now complete and dry. There will be no post-operative bruising in this area, nor is ligating the vessel required. This simple step hastens the entry into the abdomen, makes the procedure more efficient, and provides a more appealing post-surgical appearance.

Once the abdomen is opened, the urinary bladder is identified and isolated with sterile moistened laparotomy sponges. A stay suture is placed to anchor the bladder in one fixed area. Creating a cystotomy incision also causes the urinary bladder to contract and become smaller after the urine is emptied. A sterile assistant is prepared with suction to remove any urine immediately before it contaminates the surgical field. Smoke evacuation accompanies the laser incision as well. The bladder is incised in a relatively avascular area near the apex on the ventral side if possible. A 0.8 mm spot size, 12 W to 15 W CW is used to vaporize a hole in the bladder serosa and mucosa. The air forced through the hollow flexible waveguide will slightly fill the bladder when the mucosa has been ablated. At this exact moment the surgeon and assistant work together to extend the incision and avoid urine contamination as the bladder empties. The full thickness incision is continued to a length that will accommodate the entry of a suction tip. The bladder is emptied of urine and the contents of the bladder, e.g., cystic calculi, are removed and submitted for analysis. It is also important to flush saline proximally and distally to ensure that there are no remaining small urethral calculi. Post-operative radiographs should be taken to document removal of all urinary calculi.

Tumor resection, polyp removal(s), or apical diverticulum reduction require the incision with appropriate tissue margins to be continued. These tissues should be submitted for histopathology. Increasing the power delivered will speed the removal of the thick transitional cell epithelium and muscularis layers, but this also creates a great deal of plume to be evacuated. The surgeon's experience should guide the removal of tissue so that the bladder can be closed properly following the procedure.

Prior to closure the cystotomy incision is aggressively wiped free of char. The edges are clean and dry. Standard closure using monofilament absorbable suture material in an inverting pattern yields highly desirable results. The abdomen is closed routinely and the patient should recover with no post-surgical hematuria. (See Case Study 21.)

Canine Urethrostomy

Primary neoplastic disease of the urethra in dogs or cats is rare. More commonly trauma, urethral prolapse, or calculi cause obstruction of urine flow, requiring amelioration via urethrotomy. Although a common procedure, it is generally very bloody and time is consumed blotting tissues dry for better visualization. The feline perineal urethrostomy procedure was commonly employed for recurrent urethral calculi, but since the advent of low ash and urinary-acidifying diets, it is not as commonly needed. Many male dogs are likewise susceptible to urethral calculi that lodge behind the os penis after being voided from the bladder. Female dogs generally respond nicely to several months of a calculolytic diet and seldom require urethrotomy, but may require cystotomy if the dissolution attempt fails. If urethral calculi are not removed quickly, post-renal azotemia will begin its snowballing effect of diffuse metabolic derangements, eventually leading to death. The CO_2 laser aids in the speed at which relief can be delivered in this life-saving procedure.

In obstructed patients that have been stabilized, a urinary catheter is usually already in place to empty urine from the bladder. In dogs, scrotal urethrotomy is ideal because the urethra is widest and most superficial in this location. Likewise, any calculi lodged at the pelvic brim or behind the os penis are easily removed from this surgical approach. The skin incision is made with 0.4 mm spot size, 6 W to 8 W, CW SP, and any char is wiped away. The scrotum is removed, and if not already neutered, orchiectomy is performed. The surgeon palpates the obstructed area and plans the urethrotomy over the calculus. The subcutaneous tissues are gently dissected away. The retractor penis muscle is identified and displaced to one side. The indwelling urinary catheter can now be appreciated clearly through the thinned urethral mucosa. Urethrotomy is preferably performed with a 0.3 mm spot size, 2 W to 4 W, pulse mode A4–A5 (Lumenis/Accuvet, Novapulse 20 W CO_2 laser®, 15% to 20% power), superpulse repeat pulse pattern or mode P6 (20% power, repeat pulse) over the calculus, but the laser incision can also be made over the urinary catheter as long as it is not damaged. Using the repeating pulse pattern allows control over the speed and depth of the incision. If the incision is made with too much power, the catheter may be damaged or lost into the bladder. This power setting allows urethrotomy without any bleeding and also preserves the urinary catheter so it may be left in place for 24 hours after the procedure.

If urethrotomy is performed, radiographs should be examined to ensure removal of all calculi before final closure. The edges of the urethra should be gently wiped using a moistened cotton-tipped applicator to remove any char. The urethra edges are opposed using 4-0 monofilament absorbable suture material to envelop the indwelling urinary catheter. A sterile assistant can control any urethral bleeding from the suture placement by dabbing epinephrine (1:1,000) at the entry and exit points of the needle, using a sterile cotton-tipped applicator. The subcutaneous tissues and skin are closed in routine fashion after rinsing the surgical field with sterile saline and wiping away any char.

A permanent urethrostomy may need to be performed for (1) calculi that cannot be removed by flushing, (2) chronic stone formers that cannot medically be kept free of calculi, (3) strictures of the urethra resulting from one or more prior urethral surgery, or (4) severe penile trauma or when penile amputation is required. The surgeon must also create a large enough mucosal-to-skin closure to allow for some stricture of the opening in the future. The edges of the urethra should be gently wiped using a moistened cotton-tipped applicator to remove any char. The urethral mucosa edges are opposed to the skin with 3-0 or 4-0 monofilament absorbable suture material. A sterile assistant can control any urethral bleeding from the suture placement by dabbing epinephrine (1:1,000) at the entry and exit points of the needle, using a sterile cotton-tipped applicator. The laser seals capillary bleeding of the urethra when it incises, and makes the procedure cleaner and faster.

Feline Urethrostomy

The technique of choice has been described in any current veterinary surgery textbook. With a urinary catheter in place, the stabilized, anesthetized patient is in sternal recumbancy with the rectum packed off. The procedure is accomplished with a few modifications for CO_2 laser assistance. Any incision of the skin can be made with the laser using a 0.4 mm spot size, 6 W to 8 W CW SP. The fibrous attachments of the penis to the ischium should be transected with scissors; yes scissors. Avoid vaporizing the ischiocavernosus muscles or the crus of the penis with the laser since inadvertent lasing of the rectum or pelvic nerves is highly likely and hazardous. Generally, when these muscles are transected at the level of their attachments, there is little hemorrhage anyway. The penile urethra is incised over the urinary catheter on its ventral aspect to the level of the bulbourethral glands using 0.3 mm spot size, 2 W, mode A4–A5 (Lumenis/Accuvet Novapulse 20 W CO_2 laser®, 15% to 20% power), superpulse repeat pulse pattern or mode P6 (20% power, repeat pulse). Any surgeon will appreciate the control of hemorrhage immediately, since there will be no bleeding of the urethral incision. The surgeon should proceed at a pace that vaporizes the urethra in one pass, yet does not damage the indwelling urinary catheter. The urethrostomy incision is completed once the widest portion of the urethra is opened, at the level of the bulbourethral glands. The surgeon should allow enough room for eventual stricture formation. Any char is wiped away with a moistened cotton-tipped applicator. The urethra is sutured to the perineal skin using 3-0 monofilament non-absorbable suture material. A sterile assistant can control any urethral bleeding from the suture placement by dabbing epinephrine (1:1,000) at the entry and exit points of the needle, using a sterile cotton-tipped applicator. The penis is amputated with a 0.4 mm spot size, 6 W to 8 W CW, and char is removed before completing the urethrostomy skin closure.

Using a CO_2 laser in feline perineal urethrostomy provides many benefits to the patient. There is certainly diminished or negligible pain following the penile amputation. Likewise, there is no post-surgical hemorrhage from incised erectile tissue (there may be hematuria from the bladder, however). The incision is cleaner because the laser sterilizes the incision as it cuts, and the faster surgery time means less anesthetic exposure.

We also had success with a urethroplasty procedure in three cats. Each had a distal urethral obstruction. One cat had a sharp crystal lodged in the tip of the penis. A second cat had been medically treated successfully numerous times for FUS, and had severe deformities of the glans penis due to numerous traumatic catheterizations. The third cat had a stricture of the distal urethra and a fibrosed, flaccid, dysfunctional urinary bladder. Each was presented for FUS treatment from different referring veterinarians. The owners declined perineal urethrostomy. Permission was granted to perform the experimental procedure, and no promises of a favorable outcome were implied. A urinary catheter was placed prior to laser treatment. The tip of the penis was excised using 0.3 mm spot size, 5 W CW in an elliptical pattern to spatulate the urethra. This geometric shape is chosen because it will cause the new distal urethra to be wider at the opening. If a circular incision is made perpendicular to the urethra, the resulting distal urethra will have a slightly smaller diameter compared to the oblique incision. At the time of this writing, none of the three cats has had an episode of FUS for at least one year after the procedure. Further similar procedures should be performed and patients followed to ensure this procedure is safe.

Vulvoplasty

CO_2 and 980 nm diode laser energy can work well in concert for resection and removal of redundant perineal skin. These types of lasers can be a valuable tool for this type of surgery due to their ability to reduce bacterial load at the incision site based on culture-sensitivity test results that we have seen. Most perineal tissue that is inflamed and hypertrophied is also infected either superficially or in association with a deep furunculosis. The perineal skin should be retracted and evaluated for proper incision outlines. Using a CO_2 laser with a 0.4 mm spot size, 8W, PWSP 10 Hz/sec an outline is identified in two arcs around the vulva dorsally and laterally. Then the skin is incised using CO_2 laser energy with a 0.4 mm spot size 10 W CWSP. A 980 nm diode laser is then used with a 600 um fiber, 10 W CWCM (continuous wave contact mode) to excise and resect the subcutaneous fat and any granulation tissue. We have found that the diode laser provides superior incising through granulation tissue with reduced fluid volume. Make sure that sterile saline is provided as a continuous irrigation while resecting the tissue. All char is wiped clean and the incisional edges are matched up to assure adequate stretching of the perineal tissue immediately adjacent to the vulva. Then, begin skin closure by placing simple inverted interrupted monofilament absorbable sutures into the sub-Q and fascia to close the dead space. Skin closure is completed with additional monofilament non-absorbable simple interrupted skin sutures. To reduce the potential for fecal contamination or urine scald, a topical collagen coating can be used, or cyanoacrylic applied to the surface of the wound edges.

Our experience shows that the patient is very comfortable postoperatively when laser energy is used to expedite removal of the redundant perineal tissue. Rarely is an Elizabethan collar required. Topical anesthetic gel can be dispensed to further reduce any post-incisional itching or discomfort.

Vaginal Fiberoscopic Procedures

Numerous vaginal vault anomalies can be found with fiberoscopic equipment. Often, connective tissue tags, or stenosis from vaginal mucosa scarring due to some trauma, produce changes in urine flow that disrupt normal evacuation or cause pooling of the urine. Chronic low-grade infections, spotting, or dribbling of urine can often follow these tissue anomalies. Both CO_2 and diode lasers can be placed through the working channel of fiberoscopic devices. Special extended semi-flexible waveguide extensions are available to carry CO_2 laser energy to the target tissue. The vaginal vault region is typically not too moist to allow for appropriate CO_2 laser energy release to transect, bisect, or ablate redundant or adhered tissue within the vaginal vault.

Some cases require that the vaginal vault be distended with fluid to adequately see the offending tissues. Here, diode laser energy is superior because it can transect, bisect, or ablate in an aqueous environment. Grasping endoscopic forceps also are very valuable for placing tension on the tissue to be removed. This allows for more accurate, rapid, and complete removal of redundant tissue. Sutures are typically not required when resecting tissue in this area. Because of the delay in fibroblast migration after laser energy, use of a significant reduction in contracture of the vaginal tissue is noted in the immediate and mid-range post-operative period. Follow-up fiberoscopic examination in three to six weeks is critical to assure no recurrence.

Cutaneous Mass Removal

Small benign papillomas can be ablated using a 0.8 mm spot size, 6 W to 8 W CW. A local anesthetic alone can be used to remove one or two small lesions in favorable anatomic areas of cooperative patients. Larger masses require general anesthesia before removal is attempted.

Lasers provide the veterinary surgeon with unprecedented speed, accuracy, and cleanliness when removing multiple cutaneous masses. With cutaneous masses less than 0.5 cm in diameter, the wound resulting from growth removal can be left open without the need for sutures. This is accomplished by "caramelizing," or mildly charring the tissue using a defocused beam of low power intensity (e.g., 0.8 mm spot size, 4 W to 6 W CW). The resultant caramelized tissue acts as a bandage. If a scanner is available, many of these tumors can be rapidly ablated with 6 W to 10 W of power in SP mode. Scanner technology enhances laser ablation by generating a scanned laser pattern of up to 3 mm in diameter versus the standard spot size of 0.3 mm to 1.4 mm, making quicker work of ablating larger surface areas. An antibiotic ointment applied twice daily for one week will keep the healing tissues moist and encourage rapid re-epithelialization.

Any wound created with a CO_2 laser that is greater than 0.5 cm in diameter should be wiped free of char with moistened gauze, and then sutured closed. To excise these larger masses, 0.4 mm spot size, 6 W to 8 W SP is used to make an elliptical incision around the mass. Appropriately sized tissue margins are excised as well. Once the edges are defined, a 0.8 mm spot size, 10 W to 12 W CW can be used to more rapidly excise and ablate tissue by cleanly dissecting it away. When submitting the specimen for histopathology, larger tissue margins should be submitted because some shrinkage will occur due to desiccation.

The main advantage of using a CO_2 laser in these procedures is diminished post-operative pain. The hemostatic action of the laser also enhances intra-operative visualization and increases surgical speed by decreasing bleeding and the time usually spent keeping the site free of blood. Furthermore, when anesthesia is a concern due to the patient's age or other factors, less invasive laser surgery under local anesthetic provides a safer alternative. (See Case Studies 1, 3, 19.)

Lick Granuloma Therapy

Ablation of the hyperplastic granuloma complex tissue can be effectively accomplished using CO_2 laser energy. The objective is to ablate the granuloma to or just slightly below the surrounding normal dermal margins. Many of these types of granuloma lesions can be managed with local topical or injectable anesthetic agents and mild opiate restraint. General anesthesia is recommended for larger and more aggressive granuloma tissue. To provide the most effective and rapid treatment, we use a 1.4 mm spot size, 20 w CW for small granuloma lesions 1 cm or less. The laser energy is applied in a tracking linear fashion over the entire surface of the granuloma. Char is wiped away before the next pass is made. Each subsequent pass should be evaluated for depth of ablation with respect to the surrounding normal dermis. Larger granulomatous masses benefit from a mechanical pattern scanner that can provide a larger final focal spot diameter under mechanical pattern repetition. This device uses a .8 mm spot size that will allow greater power density application. A reduction of 5 W to a power level of 15 W is dialed in and the same evaluation of ablation depth observed. The addition of greater vaporization potential reduces char production. Once the granuloma is reduced, all char is removed, so it cannot act as a foreign body or nidus for bacterial growth. Then a light coating of an antibiotic cream is applied and the area wrapped with a light, soft bandage for 24 to 48 hours. The owner or the clinician can remove the bandage. The area should be rechecked in one to two weeks. Some cases require two to five treatments to completely resolve the granuloma lesion.

It is imperative to note that there are often one or more underlying etiologies with respect to a lick granuloma. A complete history of behavioral problems and complete examination for osteoarthritis and infectious or metabolic disease should be completed to assure that proper support therapy is instituted to prevent re-aggravation of the area. (See Case Studies 16a and 16b.)

Eyes

Laser-Assisted Third-Eyelid Gland (Cherry Eye) Repair

Morgan, et al. described a "pocket technique" for correcting inflamed gland nictitans as 95% successful in all breeds. This is our preferred technique as simplified with a CO_2 laser. The key advantage to using laser in this technique is hemostasis. There is an appreciable engorged conjunctival vessel that supports the gland of the nictitans. When it is transected to create the pocket that receives the tucked-in nictitans gland, a great deal of hemorrhage generally obscures the field. However, by first vaporizing this vessel with 0.3 mm spot size, 4 W CW, the posterior bulbar conjunctival incision is made clean and dry. The incision is then continued around the inflamed gland with the SP setting to minimize char. After wiping away any excessive char, the bulbar conjunctival pocket is developed by blunt dissection using iris scissors. The wound edges are opposed with 4-0 or 5-0 monofilament absorbable suture material in a continuous pattern in such a way as to tuck the gland into the developed pocket. The pocket is sealed shut by a second layer of a continuous inverting absorbable suture pattern. The tails of the suture are tied in a knot on the palpebral surface of the third eyelid. Tying the knots on the bulbar surface of the third eyelid may cause corneal trauma and should be avoided. An ophthalmic antibiotic ointment is then applied twice daily for five days. (See Case Study 27.)

Entropion Correction

Either upper or lower lid entropion can be managed quite nicely in most breeds of dog or cat. The Chinese Char-Pei, German Shepherd, Labrador Retriever, and Rottweiler have a breed predilection for this problem. If left untreated, the eyelashes continually irritate the cornea, causing epiphora, blepharospasm, corneal edema, ulceration, and in severe cases, blindness. Early intervention can produce highly desirable lifelong improvement. There are several laser surgical techniques for correcting entropion.

The ultimate goal of entropion correction is to evert the eyelids, thereby ceasing corneal irritation by the eyelashes. Laser treatment of the orbital skin and adnexa has proved useful for entropion correction in our hands. Regardless of the technique employed by the surgeon, entropion correction using CO_2 laser is generally achieved without sutures, and the results are excellent. We prefer to use a 0.4 mm tip, 2 W to 4 W CW in small dogs, and 0.8 mm spot size, 6 W to 8 W CW for large dogs. Note that at these settings the power density is below vaporization threshold. The objective is contraction of the collagen and denaturing protein at the laser tissue juncture. The beam should be held steady with the focal point on the target tissue. Only one pass is made, and it should NOT be full thickness. To achieve this, use a relatively fast hand-speed. A full thickness incision will allow relaxation of the skin covering the tarsal plate, thus defeating the purpose of the laser use in this procedure. Half thickness passes will cause permanent denaturing of collagen and connective tissue of the dermis. This desirable effect causes the skin to tighten and shorten along the longitudinal axis of the laser beam pass. This effect is immediately visible to the surgeon and "what you see is what you get" as far as the degree of change created. The pass should continue as long as the effect is noticed. When the effect stops, the surgeon should stop lasing and move on to another area.

If unsatisfactory changes have occurred with one pass, it is NOT advisable to make a second pass over the first. Instead, another pass should be made on an adjacent area, or a different technique should be employed (see below). The majority of char is very gently wiped away using a moistened gauze or moistened cotton-tipped applicator. Avoid excessive wiping that will cause irritation to the sensitive periocular tissues. The greater the experience of the surgeon, the more favorable the outcomes. CO_2 laser surgeons have used a variety of patterns, including:

- A series of "X" marks made on the skin adjacent to the lid margin, in either one or two parallel rows.
- Longitudinal streaks radiating from the lid margin and perpendicular to it.
- Char-Pei dogs may require a single pass directly on the lid margin to evert the lid in conjunction with other techniques. This breed is particularly over-represented with entropion cases, and is also particularly resistant to corrective techniques. This is due to the high mucin content in their skin that allows for the highest amount of thermal relaxation and return to a state of entropion after surgery. Full wedge resection to achieve cosmetic return to normal eyelid margin position also can be performed with the CO_2 laser.
- Scanner pulses of 100 msec to 500 msec at 4 W to 6 W CW in a pattern parallel to the lid margin, similar to the "X" marks, can be used as well, either in one or two parallel rows. This will leave a row of several 3 mm circular char deposits along the lid margin. Experienced laser surgeons may consider using continuous wave output to achieve a more rapid evertion of the eyelid margin.
- Lateral canthotomy can be performed in extreme cases to loosen up a flap of tissue. Because the laser will tighten the skin near the lid to evert

it, freeing up some tissue may enhance the appearance of the eye. Ablate the lateral canthus with 0.4 mm spot size, 2 W to 4 W CW or 0.8 mm spot size, 10 W to 12 W CW.

- In the most severe cases, a crescent-shaped wedge of tissue must be excised, and the laser can be used to make that incision. Unfortunately in these cases, fine monofilament cosmetic sutures must be placed to oppose the skin edges after undermining tissue and removing the wedge of skin.

An Elizabethan collar should be worn for two weeks to prevent self-mutilation. A recheck examination should be scheduled at that time, and if any scabs are present they can then be gently wiped away with moistened gauze. The CO_2 laser entropion correction technique is easy to perform. Anesthetic episodes are brief, and there is reduced tissue trauma from over-manipulating sensitive periocular skin and adnexa. The laser is an ideal instrument to use to correct entropion of the upper or lower lid. Nevertheless, if these procedures do not produce the desired effect and the cornea is still compromised, the patient should be referred to a veterinary ophthalmologist. (See Case Studies 14a and 14b.)

Meibomian Adenoma

The hyperplastic gland is identified at the bulbar conjunctiva of the lid. Protect the cornea by packing it off with moistened gauze. The gland may also be isolated using chelazion forceps. Vaporization of only the gland can be achieved using 0.3 spot size, 4 W, CW SP. A wedge of eyelid skin should not have to be excised to remove the entire gland. Alternately, the laser surgeon can elect to dissect the gland away from the lid using 0.3 diameter spot size, 5 W PWSP. We consider this a viable alternative because ablating the tissue will cause some peripheral heating, swelling, and possibly retention of some hyperplastic tissue. An ophthalmic antibiotic ointment is applied twice daily for five days. Sutures usually are not required with this technique.

Distichiasis and Ectopic Cilia

These tiny atypically positioned hair follicles can cause great discomfort and damage to vital external eye structures. CO_2 laser energy provides a superior alternative to more invasive scalpel incision resections.

Using a 0.3mm spot size, 5 W CW single pulse, 200 msec setting, the hair follicle is threaded up into the lumen of the laser spot tip. In cases where focusing handpieces are used, make sure the aiming beam is positioned exactly at the opening to the hair follicle. The foot pedal is then depressed three to five times in quick succession until a small grayish liquid and plume are in evidence. This indicates the bulb and associated sebaceous gland have been vaporized. The resulting laser trough will rapidly fill in with collagen over the next three to five days. A triple antibiotic ointment with or without steroids can be administered for two to three days post-operatively to reduce any mild discomfort. Patients almost never require any restrictive headgear to prevent self-mutilation.

Enucleation

Standard technique for this procedure has been described in a number of currently available surgical text books. A lateral canthotomy is performed with 0.4 mm spot size, 4 W to 6 W CW SP. The bulbar conjunctiva is dissected away from the globe using the same setting. The ocular rectus muscles are transected, freeing up the globe progressively in this process. The retrobulbar fat is dissected away to expose the optic stalk. The optic artery vein and nerve are simultaneously clamped, ligated with absorbable suture, and transected using a 0.8 mm spot size, 8 W to 10 W CW SP. For greater ease in this constricted area, use 50 mm, 90° curving tips. Following removal of the globe, the extraocular tissues are removed with traction using 0.8 spot size, 8 W to 10 W CW. The nictitans is completely removed with the same laser setting. The eyelids are removed near the eyelid margin by making a periocular pass with a 0.3 mm spot size, 3 W to 5 W CW SP or 0.4 mm spot size, 5 W to 7 W CW SP and traction. Any char is aggressively wiped away. After flushing the enucleated orbit with sterile saline, the lids are sutured closed. It is advisable to have the patient wear an Elizabethan collar until the sutures are removed to minimize self-mutilation. The use of CO_2 laser in this procedure dramatically improves the patient's post-operative comfort. There is less or no bleeding, heat, or swelling following this laser procedure. The surgeon also works much more efficiently due to the minimal time spent blotting out the normally vigorous capillary bleeding in this highly vascular area.

Laser Surgery of the Pinna and Ear Canal of the Dog and Cat

General

Dogs have a moderately higher incidence of ear disease processes than cats. Common ear ailments of dogs and cats can be seen in up to 50% of patients in areas of humid climates during some or all of the patient's life. Any disease of the ear will cause pronounced inflammation. Frequently, there is also a combination of bacterial and fungal infection in and around the ear. Any surgical procedure of the ear is therefore contaminated, painful, and hemorrhagic. Fortunately, CO_2 laser is an efficient way to manage many diseases of the ear, including proliferative otitis externa, excessive hair in the canals, aural hematoma, polyps, proliferative tumors, squamous cell carcinoma, frostbite, and trauma. The primary advantage of using laser for surgery of the inflamed ear is that hemorrhage is minimized or can be controlled. There is also reduced post-operative pain, making the use of this tool a necessity for the humane surgeon. In addition, the increased speed at which procedures can be performed benefits the patient since there is reduced anesthetic exposure.

Treating the variety of inflammatory, infectious, neoplastic, and chronic connective tissue changes that can be observed in small animal patients is often very frustrating. This is due to the small area in which the clinician has to work. It also is related to the lack of extra skin in this anatomical region or excessive inflammation to the dermis and underlying connective tissues. Recurrence or lack of complete resection of specific conditions often leads to repeated treatments, extended duration of disease processes, and increased client concern and dissatisfaction. Using laser energy can simplify the therapeutic protocol and hasten the patient's recovery.

Examination of the Ear

Examination of the pinna, ear canals, and tympanic membranes must be done in a thorough and repeatable fashion to determine the best course. In many cases the patient is uncomfortable or in outright pain from the otic condition. It is critical that the clinician take appropriate measures to ensure the patient's comfort and to fully evaluate the ear structures. Sedation using injectable medication or inhalant anesthetics is critical in most cases to perform a thorough examination of the ear canal and make the correct diagnosis. Afterward, the clinician can institute an appropriate and effective therapeutic plan.

A variety of otoscopic and otoendoscopic equipment is currently available to the practitioner. Clinicians should invest in this technology to achieve the best therapeutic outcome. Currently manufactured otoendoscopic equipment allows working channels in the body of the handpieces to transmit laser energy. Most CO_2 handpieces that use tips can be equipped with tips long enough to pass through the working channel to reach the target tissue. Silicon fibers (600 μ to 1,000 μ) are also small enough to pass through the working channel and through it, so laser energy can be delivered to the target tissue. Because ear disease contributes so much to the demands on a small animal practitioner, it is important to select equipment that effective transmits laser energy to the target tissue through otoendoscopic equipment.

The initial examination should allow the clinician to remove all of the ceruminous wax, sebaceous wax, hairs, epithelial debris, or other lumen debris from the pinna and ear canal. Any pus should be suctioned and analyzed to determine its constituents. Then this pus should also be completely removed and the ear canal thoroughly lavaged and sanitized. The otoscopic exam may be limited in certain conditions when excessive inflammatory tissue has built up. The clinician must consider if ablation of this tissue by use of laser energy will facilitate further examination. If this is not possible, more invasive techniques should be used to completely expose the ear for complete evaluation.

The normal pinna should be soft and pliable. The hair should be smooth and clean. The medial surface epithelium should be a light pink and be clean, smooth, and moderately cool to the touch.

The normal ear canal epithelium should be a light pink color. The blood vessels should be small and non-evident on casual examination. A small amount of cerumen and wax are considered normal for the healthy ear. Small amounts of hair along the vertical canal are considered normal. The horizontal canal should be routinely found to be free of hair or have a minimal number of hairs present. At the end of the horizontal ear canal, the tympanic membrane in both the dog and cat should appear as a thin translucent to transparent structure. It should be concave and have mild reflective properties. The dorsal portion of the tympanic membrane, the pars flaccida, is the opaque pink or white portion of the tympanum. It contains a network of small blood vessels. The malleus should be visible through the ventral portion of the tympanic membrane, the pars tensa. The footplate of the malleus contacts the pars tensa at the 5 o'clock position in the right ear, or the 7 o'clock position in the left ear. This is important to consider when performing laser-assisted myringotomy, and will be discussed shortly.

Initiating Causes of Ear Disease

The vertical portion of the ear begins at the tip of the pinna and continues as the ear canal, which is an invagination of epidermis forming a hollow skin tube along the inside of the head on either side. The pinna and this tube are formed by auricular cartilage, which ends in a tympanic membrane (eardrum) to identify the boundary of the external ear canal. The normal lumen is 0.5 cm to 1 cm in diameter and varies in length from 5 cm to 10 cm. Deep in the tympanic membrane lies the middle ear. This region consists of the tympanic cavity and walls, medial wall of the tympanic membrane, auditory ossicles and associated ligaments, muscles and nerves (chorda tympani and other smaller nerves), and auditory tube. The middle ear is divided into three parts: the dorsal, middle, and ventral areas. The ventral portion is the largest area. The dorsal section acts as a reservoir to trap debris and toxins. This portion has the poorest access and is difficult to adequately examine by otoscopy. Branches of the facial nerve, vagus nerve, carotid artery, and lingual artery all run close to or along channels of the middle ear.

Primary factors that initiate ear disease are those conditions of the skin that also have a direct effect on the skin that lines the pinna and ear canal. Allergic conditions, parasites, foreign bodies, keratinizing diseases, and neoplasias all can play a role in ear disease.

Certain breeds are more predisposed to diseases of the ear. These include the Shar Pei (stenotic canal), Cocker Spaniel, Laborador Retriever, Springer Spaniel (have more cerumen glands), and Poodles (excessive hair growth in the canal). Excessive trauma induced by the patient can increase ear disease. Pathological changes in the ear associated with excessive fibrosis or tumors producing fissures and deep crevices will also augment the likelihood of secondary bacterial and fungal infections.

Specific Laser Therapy Goals

Once the underlying cause of any ear disease is identified, a plan for treatment, including surgical correction using laser energy, can be formulated. Within the confined surgical space of the ear canal, the use of laser energy aids the surgeon performing procedures. CO_2 laser energy, and in some cases diode laser energy, allow for more precisely targeted ablation of tissue. A laser can simplify a number of procedures, improve near-term recovery, and provide for more normal functional anatomy. Incorporating laser surgery following thorough ear cleaning and medical therapy can treat disease components that predispose or perpetuate disease.

The first step is to determine how the energy will be applied to the target tissue. Standard laser techniques can typically be used on the pinna to accomplish the desired goals. Laser surgery of the pinna is similar to techniques used for other areas of the dermis. In the external ear canal an otoscopic or fiberoscopic otoscope can be used to facilitate visualization and direction of the laser energy. This is usually accomplished by extending the direction of the laser energy through special tips that fit into and through working channels in the otoscopic equipment. This allows the clinician to visualize the area and provide treatment within the confined space of the external ear canal.

Laser Surgery of the Pinna

The soft cartilage of the pinna generally vaporizes nicely with CO$_2$ laser energy, but higher power settings are required due to the tissue's inherent low water content. When working with the pinna, use 0.8 mm spot size, 10 W to 15 W CW. If only the skin is the target, then 0.4 mm spot size, 6 W to 8 W SP is ideal. Over the ear canals, though, first vaporize the skin, then change tips to vaporize the cartilage. Although at first a 0.4 mm tip at high power settings may seem appropriate to use for the cartilage, it will take a long time to achieve the sharp incision required to open an ear canal. Any long period of incision time will generally induce thermal conduction and thermal necrosis, and consequentially dehiscence of the final sutures. Using the larger 0.8 mm spot size will actually allow the surgeon to sharply incise the cartilage of the ear canal faster. It is important to decisively ablate the cartilage in one incisional pass to minimize char formation. Any char should be aggressively wiped away with moistened gauze. The result should be a clean and dry incision that is less painful, less hemorrhagic, and less contaminated. All of these factors contribute to a successful outcome and minimize post-surgical complications.

Benign and malignant tumors that can affect the pinna may be treated using CO$_2$ laser energy. Standard technique for resection or ablation should be used in this area with special emphasis on the conservation of normal tissue to provide functional and cosmetic results. Ablation of masses should be accomplished using a 0.8 mm spot diameter or larger, or a scanner attachment. The objective is to ablate the atypical tissue without producing peripheral tissue trauma from thermal injury. The use of power settings that provide for complete vaporization is critical in this region. Where the mass is underlying dermis and not attached, the dermis should first be incised using standard incision techniques along the parameters of a 0.4 mm spot diameter and using a power setting of at least 6 W.

A specific area of the pinna can also be effectively amputated using CO$_2$ laser energy. This technique should be used only when the mass or area of abnormal tissue cannot be effectively ablated. We have found that a 0.4 mm spot size at a power setting of 10 W efficiently incises both the dermis and the auricular cartilage. The tissue edges can then be sutured similar to ear cropping techniques or via application of surgical grade cyanoacrylic tissue adhesive.

Ear cropping procedures have also been enhanced by the use of CO_2 laser energy. The pinna can be sculpted freehand or with a surgical guide. In either case, the use of CO_2 laser energy significantly reduces the pain, swelling, and bleeding typically associated with standard scalpel technique. A spot diameter of 0.4 mm at a power setting of 10 W to 15 W produces excellent results. We have reviewed both types of closure techniques and find that tissue adhesive cyanoacrylics provided excellent closure and reduced maintenance.

Treatment of a pinna that will not stand correctly due to poor cropping technique, or a pinna that has an exaggerated curve after ear crop, is in some cases repairable using CO_2 laser energy. In this type of reconstruction the laser energy is delivered to cause a similar effect as in entropion repair. The objective is to contract the overlying dermis so that the pinna either stands up more correctly or curves less severely. To accomplish this procedure the hair should be shaved away completely over the area to be treated. A spot size of 0.8 mm or larger or a scanning attachment should be used to direct the laser energy. The power setting should be only high enough to produce collagen contraction to the dermis. Full thickness incisions should be avoided. This technique may also require rigid taping of the pinna following the therapy to ensure the underlying auricular cartilage "learns" the new position.

In cases where the pinna is badly damaged or neoplastic spread is too great, complete amputation of the pinna can be accomplished more effectively using CO_2 laser energy. Here again, the laser energy allows for more efficient removal of the pinna with less bleeding and post-operative discomfort. We recommend that after the pinna has been removed, the auricular cartilage edge be resected an additional 5 mm to allow for more complete cosmetic suturing of the skin edges.

Aural Hematoma Repair

Self-inflicted trauma is the most common cause of aural hematoma in the dog and cat. It generally arises from injury to the concave auricular cartilage and the vasculature that supports it. The source of injury is usually from vigorous and repeated head shaking or other blunt trauma. Chronic bacterial/fungal otitis externa, foreign objects in or near the ear canal, or *Otodectes sp.* infestation generally initiate intense irritation. Affected cats typically traumatize the affected ear with their own ipsilateral hind legs. Pendulous-eared dogs create the problem in the same way, or more commonly traumatize the ear against the neck and crown of the skull. One or both ears can be affected in this painful and disfiguring condition. In addition to relieving the hematoma, the underlying cause of otic irritation should be identified and resolved.

Surgeon's preference has commonly been employed in aural hematoma repair. We suggest applying the following CO_2 laser surgery concepts to your successful, established technique. The pinna is surgically prepped under general anesthesia. Using the scanner, apply 15 W CW to a single point on the concave surface of the ear hematoma near its tip to allow for drainage of fluid. Equally effective is the use of a 0.4 mm spot size, 6 W to 8 W, CW SP to produce a circular to ovoid full thickness incision to allow effective evacuation of fluid. To vaporize enough tissue to lance the hematoma, it may be necessary to use several cycles of lasing then wiping away char with a moistened cotton-tipped applicator. When most fluid has been evacuated, repeat this step on several other locations. A moistened cotton-tipped applicator can be placed through the initial incision and used as a back stop on the placement of the additional holes. Some clinicians find this to be all that is needed to produce adequate drainage for the hematoma reduction. Other clinicians may want to perform an additional step for further evacuation or in cases where excessive fibrous connective tissue has been produced. This next step is to make an incision along the length of the hematoma using the scanner setting at 10 W to 14 W CW or spot size previously discussed. The incision can be straight or sigmoidal, depending on preference. The goal is to vaporize all the skin in a 3 mm wide path, exposing the auricular cartilage but not vaporizing it. If the first pass does not achieve this, wipe away any char with gauze, then reduce the power setting and repeat the incisional pass under tension to separate the tissues efficiently.

The entire contents of the hematoma cavity can be removed once this elongated incision is made. Often fibrin clots, blood, pus, or foreign objects can be flushed out by irrigation with warm sterile saline. Mattress sutures are now placed through the ear parallel to the incision. Placing a stent on the convex surface of the ear often provides additional support to the ear as it heals slowly by contracture and re-epithelialization. A light protective bandage is applied for several days. The patient is sent home taking anti-inflammatory and broad-spectrum antibiotic medication for ten days. Sutures are removed in fourteen to twenty-one days. Weekly rechecking is advisable to ensure that the original otitis is resolving and that the hematoma repair is successful.

If a scanner is not available, this procedure may be attempted with a standard 0.8 mm tip using the same settings previously described. In cats, it may be wise to use a 0.4 mm tip 6 W to 8 W CW since feline hematomas are generally smaller and their skin is thinner. The major advantages of using laser in the treatment of this condition are clear. The patients seem to be less uncomfortable following surgery and shake their head less. There is less bleeding during the procedure and during the immediate post-operative period. Using the scanner definitely enhances this procedure since the incision that opens the hematoma cavity is actually a 3 mm skin defect. This facilitates proper drainage of the hematoma and prevents recurrence of the hematoma during the healing phase. In the feline patient we have noted considerable less pinna contracture. Using some supporting pinna wraps to act as a template for collagen healing, the feline patient does not have to end up with the marked contracture of the pinna commonly seen with scalpel techniques.

Yet another technique is to produce multiple (three to eight) small (5 mm to 15 mm) elliptical incisions through the medial skin surface of the pinna using CO_2 laser energy. A spot diameter of 0.4 mm with a power setting of 6 W to 10 W provides excellent incisions and minimizes any damage to the lateral auricular cartilage surface. CO_2 laser energy has the advantage in this case of slowing fibroblast migration across the incision area. This allows the incisions to remain open longer, facilitating better drainage. A variety of supportive suture techniques to reduce dead space have been advocated. Each individual clinician should use a technique that produces consistently positive results. Sutures have been found to be critical as a scaffold for fibroblast migration to introduce connective tissue to close down the hematoma (see Case Study 15).

Pinna-External Ear Canal Interface

This region of the ear can be easily accessed for treatment, ablation, or resection purposes. The CO_2 laser allows for efficient removal of redundant tissue, excessive granulation tissue, infected tissue, or dead tissue. We have had remarkable results in resection and ablation of excessive granulation tissue obstructing normal access to the external canal. This tissue can be ablated using a spot diameter of 0.8 mm or greater at a power setting of 12 W to 20 W. If the tissue is relatively well pedunculated, a spot diameter of 0.4 mm at a power setting of 8 W can be used to excise the tissue. The CO_2 laser has allowed for very large areas to be resected or ablated without significant discomfort to the patient after the procedure. Removal of this excessive tissue also provides for easier access to the external ear canal for application of medications or to further remove excessive granulation tissue within the canal.

External Ear Canal

Both the vertical and horizontal regions of the external ear canal can be accessed for CO_2 laser energy delivery. Standard otoscopes can be used in larger breed dogs and in areas where abnormal tissue or neoplastic tissue is not too far down the vertical ear canal. An extension tip can be attached to allow access to the atypical tissue through the otoscope-viewing channel. It is preferable, however, to use an otoendoscope for vaporization work in the external ear canal because it provides a greater range of access and visibility. Using such a device in combination with CO_2 laser energy application to targeted tissue can provide huge savings in time and reduced need for more aggressive exposure techniques.

Flexible laser delivery tips allow for the CO_2 laser energy to be directed at 10° to 90° angles to the scope. This helps to avoid unwanted damage to normal tissue or the tympanic membrane. As a reminder, CO_2 laser energy will not transmit through a fluid-filled environment, as is the case many times when performing otoendoscopy. Here, a diode laser is superior for ablation of abnormal tissue or for myringotomy. The diode laser also ablates larger sections of granulation tissue more rapidly when used in contact mode. It is very important to remind diode laser users that increased peripheral thermal tissue injury is very likely if adequate irrigation is not maintained during vaporization.

Lateral ear canal resection technique (Lacroix-Zepp) can also be greatly enhanced with CO_2 laser energy. (See Case Study 18.) CO_2 laser energy can replace standard cold steel when exposure to the horizontal canal or vertical canal is required via a lateral ear canal resection technique. There are unique benefits in CO_2 laser energy application for this technique. Bleeding, post-operative swelling, and pain have been markedly reduced for our patients. The need for extreme measures to bandage the area post-operatively is also greatly reduced.

Standard surgical protocols and anatomical landmarks for this procedure have been described. CO_2 laser energy can be applied using a spot diameter of 0.4 mm at a power setting of 10 W to 12 W. The clinician should check the rating of the tip for appropriate power setting levels. We have found that for this technique a 0.4 mm ceramic tip provided superior cutting effect through both the dermis and auricular cartilage. Standard closure techniques can then be applied. Having CO_2 laser energy available for this procedure also allows the clinician to ablate or excise excessive granulation tissue once adequate access has been gained to the horizontal or vertical ear canal. Removal of this tissue assists in irrigation or easing application of topical medical therapy following the procedure. Aeration of the ear canal also inhibits both bacterial and fungal growth.

Total ear ablation and bulla osteotomy is the recommended technique when calcification of the external ear canal and excessive granulation tissue has produced complete occlusion of the canal lumen. Here again, standard surgical protocols and anatomical landmarks recommended in various surgical textbooks should be reviewed. A spot diameter of 0.4 mm with a power setting of 8 W to 10 W is recommended to provide both adequate incisional power density and dissectional power density. The greatest advantage of CO_2 laser energy during this surgical procedure is the excellent surgical field visibility that it provides. This is due to significant reduction in bleeding during the procedure. The added visibility helps the clinician avoid sensitive nerve structures present at the junction between the external canal and the middle canal. Post-operative drainage from the surgical site has also been much less in our experience.

Myringotomy

When otitis media is suspected, but the tympanic membrane is intact, myringotomy can be done with CO_2 laser energy. The spot size should be 0.8 mm using a power setting of 8 W to 10 W on a single 200 msec or repeated 5 Hz pulse setting (duty factor 10%). Myringotomy is performed at the ventral portion of the pars tensa at the ventral most portion of the attachment of the tympanic membrane-annulus interface near the 5 o'clock or 7 o'clock position in the left or right ear, respectively. Note that performing myringotomy in these specific locations is designed to protect against inadvertent damage to the germinal epithelium overlying the manubrium of the malleus. The primary advantage to using CO_2 laser energy is that the tympanic membrane is not touched. If indicated, the introduction of a sterile 3.5 Fr tomcat catheter will not be contaminated when it is passed through the myringotomy site for bulla content sampling. The hole produced in the pars tensa using CO_2 laser energy again has the added bonus of taking longer to heal. This provides for a longer period of time for fluid drainage from the middle ear. This is critical to the proper treatment of otitis media, which is generally a highly productive exudative disease process. (See Case Study 22.)

Oro-Nasopharynx

Squamous Cell Carcinoma

Not uncommonly, white cats are affected with this erosive, disfiguring bloody anaplasm/neoplasm that tends to be aggressive and locally invasive, and may also metastasize to the regional lymph nodes and lungs. We have seen clinical cases that have included the head, nasal planum, ear tips, and/or eyelids. These are commonly affected areas because they are generally not covered by hair and are directly exposed to sunlight. If desired, the entire nasal planum can be excised with CO_2 laser. The results are generally favorable. It is important for the client to see photos of what the patient will likely appear like immediately following the procedure and in 30 days. This will allow the client not to be excessively mortified by the initial appearance of his or her pet. Using a 0.4 mm spot size, 6 W to 8 W CWSP, the affected area is carved out, taking as generous tissue margins as is practical. The nasal turbinates cannot be completely removed, so the cosmetic and realistic goals of tumor removal must be balanced to properly manage the surgical procedure. For smaller lesions, only the affected area may be ablated, thus minimizing the potentially undesirable radical appearance of a completely removed nasal planum. Any char is gently wiped away with moistened gauze. Suturing of the surrounding dermis to the exposed mucosal surface should be done carefully to minimize dead space, while allowing the nasal openings created to be maintained. Some sneezing may occur following recovery. Topical lidocaine gel can be applied following surgery to reduce local pain and irritation that may produce repeated sneezing. The owners are instructed to administer broad-spectrum antibiotics for one week, and to gently moisten the area sterile 0.9% NaCl numerous times daily during that time.

Stenotic Nares Correction

Opening stenotic nares with a CO_2 laser is a clean, easy, and highly effective procedure for allowing greater airflow through the nostrils and reducing oronasopharyngeal negative pressure. Usually bilateral and congenital, stenotic nares frequently occur in brachycephalic breeds. Affected dogs and cats produce a loud noise on inspiration, although their owners usually do not recognize this. Many affected dogs (Lhasa Apso, Old English Bulldog, Pug) also snore at night or have respiratory stridor due to an elongated soft palate. Many cats (Himalayan, Persian) also have multiple changes around the nose and eyes such as epiphora, conjunctivitis, face-fold pyoderma, and entropion. The reduced airflow through the nostrils causes the patient to require a greater inspiratory effort, which in turn creates a greater negative pressure within the oropharynx, thus exacerbating brachycephalic upper airway syndrome.

No preparation of the surgical area is required with the patient under general anesthesia. The surgeon envisions the final nasal opening as a circular conduit for airflow. To do this, a conical-wedge shaped portion of the stenotic nare is removed using a 0.3 mm spot size, 4 W to 5 W CW SP or 0.4 mm spot size, 5 W to 7 W CW SP. Continue the incision of the nostril from the philtrum to the alar fold to make the circular shape complete. To excise the redundant tissue that causes the stenosis, apply tension as the laser dissects deep into the nostril space. The anatomical continuation of the nasal passage courses caudoventromedially. Any remaining tissue in this area may also be excised until the surgeon is satisfied sufficient tissue has been removed to ameliorate the stenosis. There should be no bleeding in this highly vascular area; however, if minor hemorrhage occurs the surgeon should apply a defocused low power laser beam for hemostasis. Sutures are neither required nor indicated unless the surgeon desires to perform the standard vertical wedge resection or the horizontal wedge resection. A pleasing cosmesis will result, and the patient will breathe easier upon anesthetic recovery. This in turn reduces cardiorespiratory stress and will prolong the life of the patient, especially if performed at a young age. Antibiotics are usually not necessary, but the owners should be instructed to keep the area clean and moist for several days to prevent buildup of mucus or scabs. (See Case Study 28.)

Brachycephalic Breed Upper Airway Syndrome Correction

Old English Bulldogs commonly have many features of brachycephalic upper airway syndrome. Other popular breeds of dogs, such as the French Bulldog, Lhasa Apso, Pekingese, Pug, and Shi-Tzu, are similarly grouped. Stenotic nares and tracheal hypoplasia also may be present in many of the dogs that have this congenital complex. These dogs generally tire easily during minor exercise and have a pronounced inspiratory stridor. The negative pressures exerted upon the oropharynx during inspiration can cause these tissues to swell and further occlude the normal flow of air to the lungs. Chronically affected animals may develop secondary acquired airway restriction from everted laryngeal saccules, and terminal laryngeal collapse. To prevent a future respiratory crisis it is prudent to correct these anatomic problems in symptomatic animals when they have reached satisfactory size and age for a safe anesthetic episode.

Elongated Soft Palate Correction

This procedure requires a backstop on the laser delivery handpiece or wet gauze placed behind the soft palate to prevent inadvertent lasing of tissues in the back of the oropharynx. In sternal recumbancy the pre-medicated patient is pre-oxygenated with either propofol or pentothal prior to anesthetic induction. If ultra-short acting injectable anesthesia is not available, then inhalant anesthetics are satisfactory; however, the surgeon will need to repeatedly intubate and re-extubate to complete the procedure. A single-stay suture is placed in the distal midline of the elongated soft palate. With the tongue in a relaxed position, the surgeon makes a visual estimation of the amount of tissue to remove, or can make a low power pass on the elongated palate to mark the area to be excised. The goal is for the soft palate to conform to the shape of the epiglottis and just barely make contact with it. Using a laser-assisted uvular palatoplasty kit, 10 W to 15 W laser power is applied to the redundant tissue using the stay suture for traction. Begin at the lateral margin of the palate and vaporize tissue in a path heading to the contralateral side. It is extremely important to keep the laser beam perpendicular to the target tissue. Tangential beams are less efficient at vaporization and will cause thermal necrosis, post-operative discomfort, and potentially disastrous bleeding into vital supporting tissues (e.g., the palatine artery). After the desired tissue is excised, visual inspection confirms the soft palate rests just above the epiglottis. Sutures are neither required nor recommended.

The dog is then intubated to enhance oxygenation during recovery from the anesthetic. Perioperative broad-spectrum antibiotics and glucocorticoids are recommended. The patient should be able to eat and drink normally following complete anesthetic recovery. There should be a noticeable decrease in both respiratory effort and inspiratory stridor following the procedure. (See Case Study 11.)

Tonsillectomy

The pre-medicated patient is pre-oxygenated prior to anesthetic. An endotracheal tube is lubricated and placed comfortably. The endotracheal tube is then packed off with moistened gauze to protect it against perforation by the laser beam, which can result in a fatal flame hazard. Forceps are used to gently grasp the tonsil and slightly elevate it from its crypt. Both tonsils are excised using 0.8 mm spot size, 10 W to 15 W CW (LAUP extension without the backstop). There should be no bleeding, and the airway should be much larger following removal of both tonsils. Some minor bleeding may occur in giant breeds or when tonsils are grossly enlarged and inflamed. Direct pressure for a few minutes, cautery, a ligature, or a defocused laser beam may then be used for hemostasis. (See Case Study 4.)

Everted Laryngeal Saccule Ablation

The laryngeal saccules are usually very edematous clear to pale white bulges of tissue cranial to the vocal folds. To access this area, the patient must be anesthetized with propofol following pre-oxygenation. This is a most difficult area to reach. Smoke evacuation is tricky, and the surgeon must coordinate every move with the technician operating the plume evacuator. Fortunately, this portion of the procedure is rapid and not much smoke will be created unless the membranes are enormous. Depress the epiglottis with Allis tissue forceps and then carefully introduce the tips into the larynx. Dilate the larynx by opening the jaws to visualize the laryngeal saccules laterally. It is more effective to permanently vaporize the laryngeal saccules. It is not practical to try excising them because the working area is very deep and tight. Ablating the laryngeal saccules with a curved 120 mm long, 0.8 mm spot size tip is much more effective than trying to excise the tissues. Ablate the laryngeal saccules with 4 W to 6 W CW power during an expiration to avoid allowing the patient to inhale its own smoke. Carefully wipe away any char with a moist, cotton-tipped applicator. This technique can be difficult to accomplish for the untrained laser surgeon. It is recommended to have a complete understanding of the anatomical considerations in this area before applying laser energy.

Perineum

Anal Sacculectomy

Clinical signs of anal sac disease usually are related to scooting, bleeding, continued discomfort, and pain. Surgical intervention is needed when standard antibiotic and anti-inflammatory treatments do not resolve the condition. Anal gland material trapped under the skin causes necrosis and irritation, which leads to the perianal area becoming infected and ulcerated. A variety of surgical techniques can be used to remove the affected anal sac. We believe a modification of the open anal sacculectomy using CO_2 laser energy provides the best exposure with the least trauma to the external anal sphincter muscles.

Mosquito forceps or a grooved director is introduced through the anal gland opening into the duct of the anal sac to identify the location of the gland. It is not necessary to infuse any material to fill the gland for enhanced visualization. An incision is made in the skin overlying the inserted instrument director using 0.4 mm spot size, 6 W to 8 W CW SP. The incision is made starting from the duct opening. With the hemostat providing mild pressure to tense the skin and anal sac and the instrument used as a backstop, the incision is extended to the apex of the anal gland. Once the skin incision is complete the process is repeated to incise the overlying muscle and open the anal sac.

Once opened, the sac can be examined and evaluated for appearance and evidence of atypical tissue or texture. The margins can then be identified and grasped using a second set of sterile hemostats. The laser energy is then applied using the same settings as stated above to separate the anal sac from the attached muscle. This minimizes muscle trauma and keeps all cutting superficially directed and away from the nerve and vascular supply to the external and internal anal sphincter muscles. The anal gland is identified as a gray saccule in between the internal and external anal sphincter muscles at about 4 o'clock and 8 o'clock. They are located alongside the rectum, running 0.5 cm to 1.5 cm deep into the tissues. An Allis forceps can be used to grasp the gland and apply outward tension. A 0.8 mm spot size, using 6 W to 10 W CW is used to dissect the subcutaneous tissues away from the gland.

Caution should be used to avoid the following potential surgical errors:

- Avoid leaving any glandular material within the perineum. Remaining anal glandular epithelial cells continually produce their highly irritating secretions and cause recurrent local dermatitis.

- Avoid inadvertent lasing of the rectum to prevent infection, incontinence, and ignition of flammable colonic gases.
- Avoid aggressive dissection in areas you are not familiar with, because incontinence may occur following transection of either the caudal rectal nerve or branches of the internal pudendal nerve. Bleeding arising from many small perineal branches of the caudal rectal artery and vein also may occur. Ligation with absorbable suture material is required if the defocused low power laser, i.e., 0.8 mm spot size using 3 W to 5 W CW, cannot seal the blood vessel.

The anal sac body, neck, and duct should be removed and submitted for histopathology. The area is examined for any bleeding or remnants of anal sac tissue. The area is then lavaged using sterile 0.9% NaCl. The muscle fibers are then carefully apposed with simple interrupted absorbable monofilament sutures. A layer of subcutaneous simple interrupted absorbable monofilament suture is then applied to close the skin edges. Simple interrupted non-absorbable monofilament suture is then used to complete the closure. The patient should wear an Elizabethan collar to prevent self-mutilation, and if the patient seems very uncomfortable, ice packs will feel soothing and keep the area clean. Stool softeners may be used in patients with dyschezia or a history of firm or hard scybalae. Broad-spectrum oral antibiotics are dispensed for a period of seven to ten days. Pain relief using NSAIDS is advisable, while the use of opioids for pain relief may be contraindicated due to their propensity to cause constipation. (See Case Study 31.)

Tail Amputation

The cauda equina of dogs and cats innervates the tail, which is an important appendage for touch, balance, and communication. There is an acute awareness of sensorimotor status of this area, and, when stimulated, can cause hyperexcitability. Therefore, all serious diseases of the tail should be considered extremely painful. When required because of trauma, unresolved deformation, or tumors and their consequential diphtheritic suppuration, amputation of the tail is a humane procedure that relieves pain and eliminates sepsis. The entire tail is shaved and surgically prepped. A tourniquet is not required. A dorsal and a ventral skin incision is made using a 0.4 mm spot size, 6 W to 8 W CW SP. The incisions are made in the shape of a "V" so that the posterior edge of the incision is pointed, and the proximal edges of the incision meet at the level of the intended separation of caudal vertebrae. Any char is aggressively wiped away with moistened sterile gauze. The surgeon must clearly identify the joint to be dissected. We use a sterile 25 gauge needle to demonstrate the intervertebral space. Under tension, vaporize connective tissue, ligaments, artery vein, and nerve at the level of the joint using 0.8 mm spot size, 6 W to 10 W CW. Avoid charring the distal edge of the remaining vertebra. The incision is lavaged with sterile saline prior to closure. Leave a small amount of skin for cushioning and closure using absorbable suture material. Do not leave an excessive remnant of redundant skin, because this may lead to seroma formation. Any excess tissue can be trimmed away prior to closure. Antibiotics are dispensed for ten days. Sutures are not required, and Nexaband S/C® may be used on the skin edges. (See Case Study 26.)

Perianal Adenoma

These lesions are common in the mature dog and should not be overlooked. Although the majority of these growths are benign, the occasional adenocarcinoma can be identified and removed early. The anus and rectum are evacuated and packed with moistened gauze to prevent escape of potentially flammable gases. A single lesion can be ablated using 0.8 mm spot size, 8 W to 10 W CW. Larger lesions require a 0.4 mm spot size, 6 W to 8 W CW SP to define the margins of the skin incision followed by vaporization of the underlying subcutaneous tissues. The lesions are then ablated using traction and a 0.8 mm spot size, with 8 W to 10 W CW power. The lesion is always submitted for histopathology. The skin edges are aggressively wiped free of char with moistened gauze, and the skin is closed routinely. With larger mass removals it may be desirable to have the patient wear an Elizabethan collar to prevent self-mutilation. Broad-spectrum antibiotics are dispensed since this anatomical area is generally contaminated

Digits

Toenail Lasing

This value-added service can be employed when dogs are anesthetized for other elective procedures. Generally, these patients have grossly overgrown toenail lengths, and the "quick" or blood vessel within the nail has grown out to the distal tip of the nail as well. This is common in the Doberman Pinscher, Rottweiler, Poodle, German Shepherd, German Shorthaired Pointer, Labrador Retriever, Golden Retriever, and Char-Pei dogs, for example. Typically these patients stressfully object to having their feet touched and may not receive the proper care they require. Lengthy toenails may split and become painfully infected or tear off or cause injury to others. It is often a concern to trim these nails back far enough so that they stay short for a long enough period of time to warrant exposure to sedation or anesthesia. Trimming the toenails back far enough to cause them to bleed quickly also requires the use of a styptic medication to speed the rate of coagulation within the nail. Unfortunately, this predisposes the patient to septic onychitis.

Using the laser in this situation is a unique solution to many of these problems. With a patient under general anesthesia or deep sedation, the toenail is trimmed back to the desired length. Using a 0.8 mm spot size at 6 W to 8 W CW or a 1.4 mm spot size at 10 W CW, the laser beam is directed toward the bleeding toenail vessel and held approximately 1 cm from the target surface. We generally employ a circular pattern from the outside toward the center to slowly cauterize the vessels and achieve hemostasis. It is important to be slightly defocused to prevent recurrent transection of the blood vessel while making these passes with the laser beam. Do not attempt to wipe away any of the protective char. Polishing with a hand-held rotary tool finishes off this technique nicely. The end result is a sterile field that is dry and smooth.

Alternately, we have found that a 0.4 mm spot diameter can be used with 10 W to 15 W CW SP at a 90° angle to the nail at the desired resection level. The nail is first moistened with sterile 0.9% NaCl for one to two minutes to increase its water component. The CO_2 laser energy is then applied in a steady single pass with some tension on the tip of the nail. This facilitates opening of the incision for subsequent passes if necessary. The newer ceramic tips allow for the higher wattage settings, which provides clean nail bisection with little or no bleeding. If small bleeding is noted from the digital vessel the CO_2 laser beam can be defocused and applied in single pulses on the bleeding vessel as mentioned in the previous example. The nail can then be polished with a rotary tool to smooth the cut edges.

Digital Amputation

Tumors of skin, bone, or connective tissue frequently affect the digit. A thorough pre-operative examination of the patient should include at minimum a biochemical profile and radiographs of the affected digit and the chest. Begin the amputation with a skin incision made with a 0.4 mm spot size, 6 W to 8 W CW SP without a tourniquet. Any char on the skin is aggressively wiped away. The incision must extend proximal to and include the associated digital pad. Switching to a 0.8 mm spot size facilitates the amputation. Using 12 W to 15 W CW, the supporting ligaments and tendons of the digit are transected at the level of the joint proximal to the diseased bone. The digital arteries, veins, and nerves are sealed as the amputation continues very similar to feline declaw procedure. Note that these vessels are somewhat larger than in the feline patient. Vessels greater than 0.6 mm may require separate ligation, the use of 980 nm diode energy in contact mode, or electrocautery to stop bleeding. After a rinse with sterile saline and removal of any excessive char, the wound is sutured closed according to the surgeon's preference. A light bandage is applied over the foot to prevent gross contamination post-op. Broad-spectrum antibiotics should be administered for one week following the procedure to prevent infection of the surgical site. The patient will feel immediate relief and the end result is cosmetically pleasing. (See Case Study 8.)

Feline Onychectomy

Feline onychectomy has been taught in veterinary colleges for many years. The first technique was the use of surgical scalpel blades, which were used to provide a more exact anatomical disarticulation of P3 while producing less tissue trauma. A variety of toenail trimmers to disarticulate P3 from the digit also have been used; disadvantages include crushing trauma to the soft tissue and failure in some cases to completely remove all of P3. Either technique was done through a dorsal approach and required a tourniquet and bandaging of the forepaws for twenty-four to forty-eight hours post-operatively. The patients were in many cases very stressed and uncomfortable for several days to weeks following this procedure.

When elective feline declaw must be done for the owner's benefit, the CO_2 laser is a superior disarticulation tool. We fully believe that CO_2 laser use for this procedure is the most humane technique. It significantly reduces post-operative bleeding, pain, and swelling, providing a quicker return to normal activities. No tourniquets or bandaging are needed, further reducing the physical and mental stress to the feline patient. Many clinicians over the past ten years have reported this technique with a variety of slight variations.[1,2]

After careful client counseling, the cat is induced with general anesthetic agents that include an opioid as well as a sedative. This provides for a very quiet and uneventful recovery from maintenance inhalant anesthesia. The success of this procedure largely depends on the experience and skill level of the laser surgeon. One preference is to trim the pointed toenails before pre-surgical cleansing. All toes are cleansed with a dilute chlorhexidine solution, and then rinsed with sterile saline. A tourniquet is not required and may be contraindicated because it causes anoxia and reperfusion injury to the tissues of the antebrachium and digits. Oschner (rat-toothed) hemostats are used to clamp P3 just proximal to the ungual crest. To dissect P3 cleanly from P2, the technique is as follows: a single laser pass with rapid hand speed using a 0.4 mm spot size, 5 W to 6 W CW is performed on the lateral surface of the ungual crest from dorsal to ventral. A similar single laser pass immediately follows on the medial surface of the ungual crest so that the two incisions meet at its dorsal-most point. If necessary, a small burst of laser energy can be used to connect the two incisions dorsally or ventrally. All laser bisections are done through a window produced by an incision through the skin overlying the annular ligament and dorsal aspect of the joint capsule. Be cautious not to overuse the laser during this procedure because the resulting excessive char formation will impair healing and cause irritation that defeats the benefits of laser declaw procedure. The thin skin covering P3 can now be advanced proximally (pushed back) to better expose the distal interphalangeal joint.

To continue the procedure, the Oschner forceps holding P3 is rotated to flex the joint. With the laser tip pointed away from P2 to avoid inadvertent charring of the remaining phalanx, the laser makes a single pass over the dorsal elastic ligament and extensor tendon and transects it using 0.4 mm spot size, 6 W to 8 W CW. It is important to continually flex P3 while applying laser energy to cause separation of P3 from P2 as previously noted. Some surgeons have found it is easier to perform this technique with the angled handpiece used so frequently in the oral cavity. It is also advisable to make clean passes with the laser and avoid going back and forth over the same area.

Excessive lasing of charred tissue will cause undesirable heating of tissues and result in post-operative pain and swelling. While continuing to laser cut the lateral collateral, then medial collateral distal interphalangeal ligaments, the surgeon should continually flex the joint to ensure that enough tension is applied to separate P3 from P2. At this point the distal inter-phalangeal joint should be completely exposed. In a final aggressive flexing maneuver, the laser is directed distally toward the backside of P3 to vaporize the deep digital flexor tendon attachment from the flexor process of P3. Note that the superficial flexor tendon bifurcates before this area and inserts on the distal aspect of P2. The laser beam can now be directed onto P3, which is being removed with tension, and should help in completely avoiding P2. The digital pad should also remain completely intact due to the aggressive flexing action during the amputation. A hole that is clean and dry will measure 2 mm to 3 mm in diameter if this procedure is followed correctly. Defocusing the beam and applying a short burst of laser energy onto any culprit vessel can control any minor bleeding.

It is essential that all of P3 be removed and that P2 not be charred during the laser declaw procedure. Any char on the skin incision is wiped away with sterile moistened gauze, and then dried with sterile gauze. Last, a small amount of tissue adhesive is applied to the skin edges only, and then sealed closed. Avoid using excessive amounts of this bonding agent, which can lead to postoperative inflammation, granulation tissue, and discomfort. It is preferable to shape the toes to a natural and pleasing appearance. Following five to ten seconds of gentle pressure, the surgical site is examined for any problems before moving on to the next toe. An injectable broad-spectrum antibiotic may be administered, and the patient is sent home with shredded paper to use as litterbox liner. Bandaging of the feet is not required. The patient should recover normally and walk comfortably. It is wise to allow the cat several days to adjust to its "new shoes," and although not painful, the cat will need to learn to walk and support weight slightly differently.

Buprenorphine or Meloxicam can be supplied in separate syringes for oral administration for the first two to three days post-operatively. It is critical that the clinician impress upon the owner the need to maintain good confinement of the cat for the first three to five days. This is particularly important because the significant reduction in pain will allow the cat to feel that it can return to its normal habits immediately. (See Case Studies 7a and 7b.)

Orthopedic/Musculoskeletal

Repair of Anterior Cruciate Ligament Insufficiency

Tibial plateau leveling osteotomy (TPLO) has enjoyed recent fame as a superior technique compared to placement of a lateral imbricating suture. The CO_2 laser cannot cut bone as required in TPLO, but may be used to diminish any pain stimuli originating from a skin incision over the stifle in any dog that requires this technique. When the lateral imbricating suture technique is elected to repair an ACL rupture, our technique is as follows: Skin and subcutaneous tissue of the left stifle is incised using a 0.4 mm spot size, with 8 W to 10 W CW SP. The medial or lateral joint capsule is identified and a small window is created in it with 0.3mm spot size, 5 W CW. Adson forceps are introduced into the joint and tent the capsule up. The laser is used to incise the capsule over the forceps using the same power setting. Any char is aggressively wiped away as synovial fluid escapes the joint. Avoid introducing any char or other foreign material into the stifle. The trochlea and patella should be examined for osteophytes. The menisci should be examined for any tears, and released if present. The remnants of the anterior cruciate ligament are ablated with a 0.8 mm EC tip (Lumenis/Accuvet), 12 W to 15 W CW. Any extremely irritating char is aggressively wiped back with a sterile moistened cotton-tipped applicator.

The capsule is then closed with 3-0 monofilament absorbable suture material. A small hole is then drilled through the tibial tuberosity to later receive the imbricating suture. The lateral fabella is clearly palpated following dissection of the overlying subcutaneous tissues with 0.8 mm spot size, 12 W to 15 W CW. A lateral imbricating suture (#2 gauge) is passed behind the lateral fabella within the femorofabellar ligament, then underneath the patellar tendon, through the tibial tuberosity, and a knot is then tied. There should be free range of motion, no crepitation, and good joint stability following the procedure. Routine skin closure is applied, followed by a support bandage.

Anesthetic recovery may include administration of opioid analgesics, although it may not be necessary due to the diminished post-operative pain experienced by patients undergoing laser-assisted ACL repair. The owner should be instructed several times to REST his or her dog, keep the bandage clean and perfectly dry, and return in ten to fourteen days for suture removal. Carprofen may be dispensed if necessary. Antibiotics should not be necessary unless body temperature rises above 103°F. The patient should recover fully if confined for ten days, strictly rested for one month, and has limited activity for three months. The use of CO_2 laser in this procedure dramatically improves the patient's post-operative comfort. Although all phases of surgical involvement cause pain due to stimulation of nociceptors, these stimuli are diminished when CO_2 laser energy seals nerve endings, blood vessels, and lymphatics during surgical incisions. Less or no bleeding, heat, or swelling all mean less pain following laser surgery. Patients can be fully ambulatory and comfortable following laser-assisted orthopedic surgery.

Pelvic and Thoracic Limb Amputations

The CO_2 laser improves visualization of anatomical dissection during amputation by improved hemostatis at the surgical site. The CO_2 laser can be used for all aspects of incisional work during amputations, including skin incision, fascial plane dissection, muscle belly transection, and nerve/vessel transectioning. The CO_2 laser is not appropriate for bisection of the bone. It is highly effective in joint disarticulations. We use both 0.4 mm spot diameters and 0.8 mm spot diameters to complete the amputations. Energy input is usually in the 10 W to 15 W range when using the 0.4 mm spot diameter and 15 W to 20 W range when using the 0.8 mm spot size. Tension on the muscle bellies being transected improves separation. Our

179

experience with post-operative recovery subjectively appears to show more comfortable patients with decreased pain, swelling, and bleeding from the incisional stump.

Endocrine

Thyroidectomy

Treatment options for the hyperthyroid cat include radioiodine therapy, daily oral anti-thyroid medicines, and surgical removal of the gland. Many owners may not wish to isolate their pet following administration of radioactive iodine. Other cats cannot tolerate daily medications required to suppress production of thyroid hormone. Surgical excision is a relatively easy procedure to perform and can be curative.

A ventral midline skin incision is made just caudal to the larynx using 0.3 mm spot size, 4 W to 5 W CW SP. Any char is aggressively wiped away. The sternocephalicus muscle is incised along its midline and retracted to expose the sternohyoideus muscle. Caution should be employed in this area due to numerous vital structures in the vicinity. The sternohyoideus is incised along its midline, exposing the trachea. Gentle traction allows identification of the enlarged thyroid lobe(s) located adjacent to the trachea, just caudal to the larynx, and medial to either vagosympathetic trunk. The caudal thyroid vein is located and isolated using forceps and a moistened sterile cotton-tipped applicator. Once the underlying structures are identified and protected, the vessel is transected and sealed with the laser using 0.3 mm spot size, 4 W CW. The surgeon must clearly identify and protect the parathyroid gland before removing the thyroid lobe.

Based on the location of the parathyroid, and the size and shape of the thyroid lobe, the surgeon must decide on performing an extracapsular or an intracapsular thyroidectomy. Either technique is acceptable, with the goal of complete thyroid lobe removal with minimal disturbance of the parathyroid gland. Care must also be taken to avoid excessive disturbance of the cranial thyroid artery because vasospasm will cause the parathyroid to necrose and predispose the cat to hypocalcemia, especially if a bilateral thyroidectomy is required. Sterile moistened cotton-tipped applicators are used to very gently tease the thyroid lobe free from its connective tissue attachments. The thyroid lobe is completely removed with 0.3 mm spot size, 4 W CW; gentle traction will facilitate separation of the thyroid from the parathyroid gland.

The specimen(s) should be submitted for histopathology. The surgeon must have very precise aim to avoid charring the parathyroid gland or injuring the cranial thyroid artery. Alternatively, one parathyroid gland can be planted within a pocket created in the sternohyoideus muscle. The muscle layers are closed with 4-0 monofilament absorbable suture material, and the skin is closed with Nexaband S/C®. If bilateral thyroidectomy is performed it is advisable to stage the procedures thirty days apart to minimize the potential for hypoparathyroidism. This technique is performed faster with a CO_2 laser because there is little or no bleeding at all during the procedure. Vaporizing the pertinent vessels obviates the need to ligate vessels, making the surgeon's time efficient, and minimizes the anesthetic exposure time to a geriatric cat. Because there is less swelling and less bleeding using the laser, the surgical site is cleaner. Therefore, the laser-assisted thyroidectomy procedure is much safer because the enhanced visibility prevents inadvertent disruption of vital structures. (See Case Study 25.)

Gastrointestinal Tract Applications

We have used CO_2 laser energy very effectively in various gastrointestinal tract procedures, including enterotomy, gastrotomy, pyloroplasty, tumor resection, lymph node biopsy, intestinal biopsy, and resection. The CO_2 laser can be used for the primary abdominal skin incision and abdominal linea alba, then in place of the scalpel for incisive and biopsy work on the GI tract. The mucosal surface of the intestinal tract is highly vascular and seals over rapidly upon closure. As always, appropriate power density is needed to reduce any potential for peripheral tissue thermal injury. Standard suture technique is applied to provide incisional apposition. There is reduced bleeding and reduced need for electrocautery application when the CO_2 is used. It is important to milk any fluid or gas out of the surgical site to avoid the potential for combustion. This has never been a complicating factor for us, but it must always be considered when using CO_2 laser energy in this region of the body, just as when working around the rectum.

Conclusion

Veterinary CO_2 laser surgery equipment provides a general practitioner with the instrumentation for dramatically improved post-operative outcomes. This equipment is now more affordable, easier to use, and is in great demand by clients. The techniques described here are our preference for elective procedures. The settings that have been discussed are only examples of the typical power settings required to accomplish the surgical task. To achieve excellent post-surgical outcomes it is important to possess a mastery of anatomy, surgical experience, and advanced training. The application of a surgical laser does not guarantee success, but its judicious use will certainly improve surgical results.

After considering the different types of laser delivery systems available to veterinary medical care providers, it is clear that the CO_2 laser is the most sensible choice for small animal practice. Furthermore, surgeons should promote more compassionate post-surgical care by diminishing the pain, swelling, and bleeding associated with most procedures. The CO_2 laser is the ideal surgical tool to expand a veterinary practice's capabilities, and it is easy to acquire the proper skills to master its use. Incorporating a laser into a practice provides additional opportunities for surgical services that can be offered to clients. The general public definitely perceives this as the highest level of quality care and they demand it.

Every day, more veterinarians are beginning to manage challenging surgical cases in their own practices without the need to outsource the labor. Practitioners who use this technology are enjoying the excitement of the nearly effortless solutions that a CO_2 laser offers to problems that previously were not as easily managed. In addition, many common procedures now performed with a CO_2 laser result in improved surgical outcomes unequalled by any other single surgical technology available to the veterinary profession. The result is happier pets and clients, improved job satisfaction to all employees of a veterinary practice, and increased practice revenue. Laser surgery is certainly here to stay, and prudent practitioners will avail themselves of its benefits.

Notes

1. Cavanaugh, Medco Forum, 1998, Vol 5, Number 1, pp 1-4.
2. Young, Vet Clinics Small Animal, 2002, pp 602-610.

Case Studies

Case Study 1
Sebaceous Adenoma of Eyelid Margin

8-year-old male neutered Retriever, presented for surgical removal of small lower right eyelid margin sebaceous adenoma.

PROCEDURE: Ablation of mass and underlying sebaceous tissue from eyelid margin (Figure CS1-1).

ANESTHESIA: Pre-medicated with medetomedine, butorphanol, and glycopyrrolate. Mask induction with isoflurane in oxygen. Maintenance of general anesthesia via endotracheal tube.

EQUIPMENT: 20-Watt CO_2 Novapulse™ laser with straight handpiece and 0.8 mm ceramic tip.

LASER SETTINGS:
    Spot Diameter: 0.8 mm
    Power Output: 10 to 15 W
    Beam Output: CW and SP

TECHNIQUE: Using the 0.8 mm tip, directed perpendicular to the mass, CO_2 laser energy is directed into the mass, ablating it completely. Sterile 0.9% NaCl is flushed into the resulting laser trough and all char removed. The resulting tissue defect (Figure CS1-2) granulates in by secondary intention.

COMMENTS: Frequent lavage and removal of carbonized debris provides good visualization of any sebaceous tissue remnants. This technique also reduces peripheral tissue heating and minimizes scarring.

CLOSURE: None. A water-based ophthalmic antibiotic ointment is applied to the site twice daily to encourage clean re-epithelialization.

POST-OP EVALUATION: Resolution of the laser trough should be complete within fourteen to twenty-one days of procedure (Figure CS1-3). Little or no scarring is noted.

FOLLOW-UP: Eyelid margin should be evaluated after seven days for evidence of proper healing, and again at six weeks to determine if complete resolution of mass has been achieved.

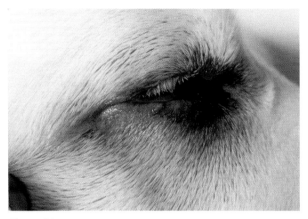

Figure CS1-1

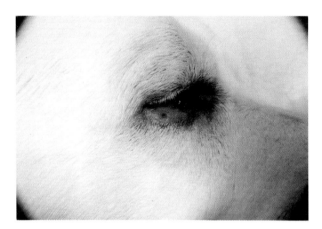

Figure CS1-2

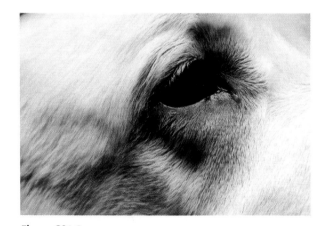

Figure CS1-3

Case Study 2
Ulcerated Sebaceous Adenoma

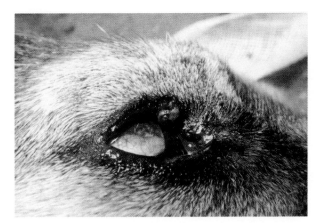

Figure CS2-1

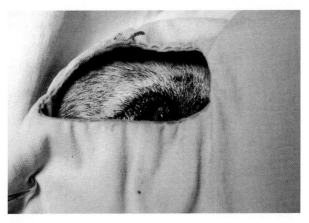

Figure CS2-2

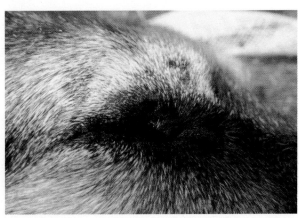

Figure CS2-3

12-year-old female Beagle, presented for removal of an ulcerated mass on the right upper eyelid margin (Figure CS2-1).

PROCEDURE: Resection of mass, minimizing loss of eyelid margin and maximizing clean tissue margins.

ANESTHESIA: Pre-medicated with medetomedine, butorphanol, and glycopyrrolate. Mask induction with isoflurane in oxygen. Maintenance of general anesthesia via endotracheal tube.

EQUIPMENT: 20-Watt CO_2 Novapulse™ laser with straight handpiece and 0.3 mm metal tip.

LASER SETTINGS:
  Spot Diameter: 0.3 mm
  Power Output: 4 to 6 W
  Beam Output: SP

TECHNIQUE: Using the 0.3 mm tip directed perpendicular to the tissue, an elliptical incision is made around the mass with care taken to minimize eyelid margin loss (Figure CS2-2). The surgical margins are lavaged with sterile 0.9% NaCl and sterile gauze sponges to remove any char. Surgical margins are evaluated for any gross evidence of any remaining atypical tissue. Surgical margins are then apposed to assure adequate tissue for primary closure.

COMMENTS: Care should be taken to protect the cornea. When the eyelid margin is involved in surgical procedures like these, minimization or elimination of peripheral tissue interaction is imperative. Adequate power density must be maintained to assure viable tissue is protected from peripheral heating. No char should be left along the incision margins prior to closure. The neoplasm should be submitted for histopathology.

CLOSURE: Two-layer closure is recommended in this case. Underlying conjunctival tissue is closed using 4-0 absorbable monofilament (Figure CS2-3). Skin is closed using a 4-0 non-absorbable monofilament. Care should be taken to avoid exposure of the cornea to suture material.

POST-OP EVALUATION: Closed incision should be evaluated at forty-eight hours and client informed to monitor patient for any signs of irritation to the incision or cornea.

FOLLOW-UP: Sutures should be removed in ten to fourteen days, providing adequate incisional healing has taken place. Conjunctival surface should also be monitored for evidence of normal healing.

Case Study 3
Canine Sebaceous Gland Adenoma Removal

10-year-old male neutered Retriever, presented for open, draining mass in dorsal cervical region.

PROCEDURE: Removal of mass.

ANESTHESIA: Pre-medicated with medetomedine, butorphanol, and glycopyrrolate. Mask induction with isoflurane in oxygen. Maintenance of general anesthesia via endotracheal tube.

EQUIPMENT: 20-Watt CO_2 Novapulse™ laser with straight handpiece and 0.4 mm metal tip.

LASER SETTINGS:
    Spot Diameter: 0.4 mm
    Power Output: 8 to 10 W
    Beam Output: SP incision, CW excision

TECHNIQUE: Using the 0.4 mm tip directed perpendicular to the tissue, an elliptical incision is made in SP mode with a single pass around the mass (Figure CS3-1). Once the skin has been incised the beam output is altered to CW to increase coagulation of tiny blood vessels during the rest of the procedure. The mass is elevated and excised by ablating the surrounding subcutaneous tissue (Figure CS3-2). Once the mass is removed, the incision and tissue defect is lavaged with sterile 0.9% NaCl and char is removed with sterile gauze sponges. Incisional margins are then apposed to assure primary intention healing.

COMMENTS: Care should be taken to provide adequate tissue margins free of tumor. Adequate power density should be maintained at all times to minimize peripheral thermal tissue damage. No char should be left in the wound after tumor excision. The mass should be submitted for histopathologic evaluation.

CLOSURE: Two-layer closure is recommended in this case. Underlying subcutaneous tissue and dead space should be closed using 2-0 absorbable monofilament suture material. Skin is closed using 2-0 non-absorbable monofilament suture material (Figure CS3-3).

POST-OP EVALUATION: Closed incision should be monitored by the client, and any swelling, redness, or fluid leakage at the incision site reported.

FOLLOW-UP: Incision should be reevaluated at ten to fourteen days. The sutures should be removed at this time as long as adequate healing has taken place and the tensile strength of the suture line is adequate. No further follow-up care should be required.

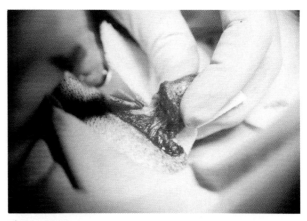

Figure CS3-1

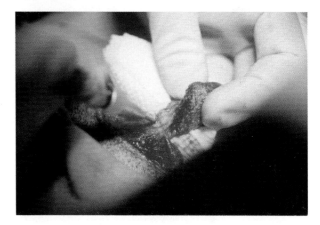

Figure CS3-2

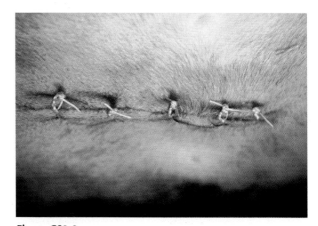

Figure CS3-3

Case Study 4
Tonsilar Carcinoma Canine

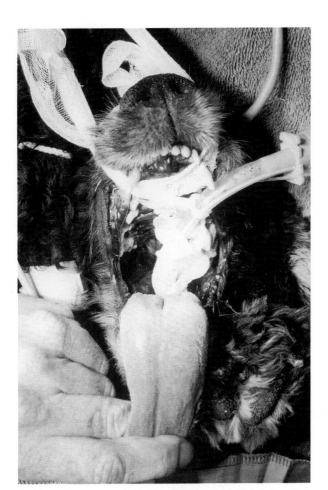

Figure CS4-1

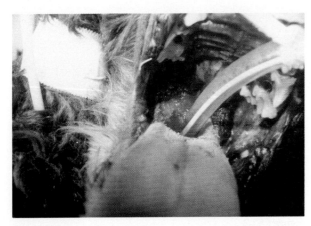

Figure CS4-2

8-year-old male neutered Norwegian Elkhound, presented for chronic halitosis and mild bleeding from the oral cavity. Oral exam revealed an everted and ulcerated right tonsil (Figure CS4-1 and Figure CS4-2).

PROCEDURE: Tonsillectomy for evaluation of potential neoplasia. Emphasis on wide tissue margin is critical for histopathology.

ANESTHESIA: Pre-medicated with medetomedine, butorphanol, and glycopyrrolate. Mask induction with isoflurane in oxygen. Maintenance of general anesthesia via endotracheal tube.

EQUIPMENT: 20-Watt CO_2 Novapulse™ laser with straight handpiece and 50 mm, 0.8 mm diameter metal tip.

LASER SETTINGS:
  Spot Diameter: 0.8 mm
  Power Output: 10 to 12 W
  Beam Output: CWNSP

TECHNIQUE: The tonsil is grasped using Allis tissue forceps and completely everted from its crypt. The surgical area is packed off with sterile 0.9% NaCl-soaked gauze sponges to protect both adjacent tissues and the endotracheal tube. The base of the tonsil is then clamped as far from the glandular tissue as possible (Figure CS4-3). The 0.8 mm tip is directed perpendicular to the tissue on the medial aspect of the forceps. The beam is directed parallel to the edge of the forceps. The tonsil is excised (Figure CS4-4) and submitted for histopathologic evaluation (Figure CS4-5). The stump is allowed to slip back into the crypt. It is evaluated for any bleeding. The area is then wiped down with a sterile 0.9% NaCl-soaked gauze sponge to remove any char. The area is examined for two to four minutes for any sign of bleeding from the stump.

COMMENTS: Care should be taken to provide adequate tissue margins of representative normal tissue. The larger spot diameter and lower PD provides for adequate vaporization with superior cauterization at the stump. Post-operative bleeding is not seen.

CLOSURE: The tonsillar fold can be sutured over using 3-0 absorbable monofilament or left open to granulate in by secondary intent (Figure CS4-6).

POST-OP EVALUATION: The surgical area should be monitored for swelling or airflow obstruction upon extubation. Owner should be informed to observe for normal eating and drinking within twelve hours of procedure. Any bleeding or other oral discharge should be communicated to the clinician.

FOLLOW-UP: Histopathology revealed a squamous cell carcinoma infiltrate in the tissue submitted. Tissue margins were free of tumor. Case was referred to veterinary oncologist for chemotherapy. Surgical site healed uneventfully.

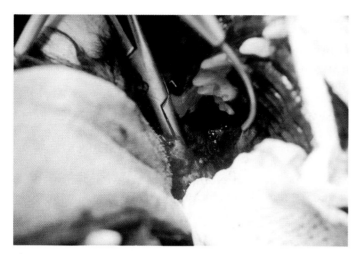

Figure CS4-3

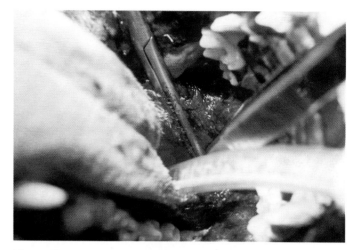

Figure CS4-4

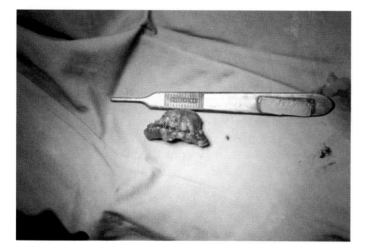

Figure CS4-5

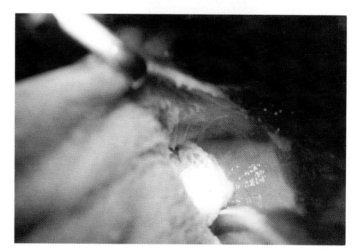

Figure CS4-6

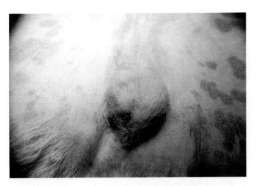

Figure CS5-1

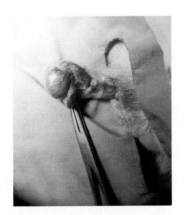

Figure CS5-2

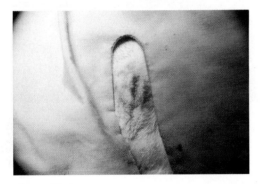

Figure CS5-3

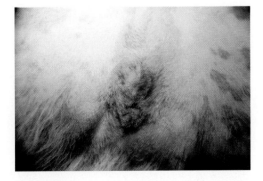

Figure CS5-4

Case Study 5
Canine Scrotal Castration

10-week-old male Argentine Dogo, presented for scrotal castration.

PROCEDURE: Single midline scrotal incision, exteriorization of both testicles, and ligation of spermatic cord, artery, and vein through this incision.

ANESTHESIA: Pre-medicated with medetomedine, butorphanol, and glycopyrrolate. Mask induction with isoflurane in oxygen. Maintenance of general anesthesia via endotracheal tube.

EQUIPMENT: 20-Watt CO_2 Novapulse™ laser with straight handpiece and 0.4 mm diameter metal tip.

LASER SETTINGS:
Spot Diameter: 0.4 mm
Power Output: 6 to 8 W
Beam Output: CWSP scrotal incision, CWNSP bisection

TECHNIQUE: A scrotal skin incision is made along median rafé (Figure CS5-1). The testes are pushed upward, causing the scrotum to be tense. The 0.4 mm tip is directed perpendicular to the targeted surgical site. The testes are pushed up and through a single incision. An incision is made into the subcutaneous tissue and spermatic fascia over each testicle using the CO_2 laser in CW mode. The tunics and associated cremaster muscle are also separated from the rest of the spermatic cord using the CO_2 laser in CW mode (Figure CS5-2). The spermatic cord, artery, and vein are transfixed using a 0 to 2-0 absorbable suture.

COMMENTS: The CO_2 laser should be used to incise, divide, and transect all tissues. This minimizes tissue handling and trauma to the tissue. There is also a significant reduction in bleeding from the skin and pain from transected nerves.

CLOSURE: The subcutis is closed using 3-0 absorbable suture material (Figure CS5-3). Clear cyanoacrylic tissue adhesive is applied to the skin edges to complete the technique (Figure CS5-4).

POST-OP EVALUATION: The patient should not lick or chew at the area.

FOLLOW-UP: The patient is re-evaluated at seven to ten days to ensure adequate healing of the skin incision and no swelling of the scrotum.

Case Study 6
Feline Scrotal Castration

16-weekold male Domestic Shorthair, presented for scrotal castration.

PROCEDURE: Single midline scrotal incision, exteriorization of both testicles through single scrotal incision with ligation of spermatic cord, artery, and vein.

ANESTHESIA: Pre-medicated with medetomedine, butorphanol, and glycopyrrolate. Mask induction with isoflurane in oxygen. Maintenance of general anesthesia via endotracheal tube.

EQUIPMENT: 20-Watt CO_2 Novapulse™ laser with straight handpiece and 0.4 mm diameter metal tip.

LASER SETTINGS:
 Spot Diameter: 0.4 mm
 Power Output: 6 W
 Beam Output: CWSP scrotal incision, CWNSP bisection

TECHNIQUE: A scrotal skin incision is made along or perpendicular to (Figure CS6-1) the median rafe' of the scrotum. The testes are pushed upward, causing the scrotum to be tense. The 0.4 mm tip is directed perpendicular to the median rafe'. The testes are pushed up to the skin incision. An incision is made into the subcutaneous tissue and spermatic fascia and tunic of the testes using the CO_2 laser in CW mode. The testes are exposed in an open tunic approach (Figure CS6-2). The tunics and associated cremaster muscle are separated from the rest of the spermatic structure using the CO_2 laser in CW mode with the tissue under tension. No clamping is required. The ductus deferens and spermatic vessels are used to tie two square knots in the spermatic cord (Figure CS6-3). The spermatic cord is transected distal to the square using the CO_2 laser in CW mode.

COMMENTS: The CO_2 laser should be used to incise, separate, and transect all tissues. No crushing of tissue is needed. This minimizes tissue handling and trauma. Significant reduction in bleeding from the skin and tunic are also appreciated.

CLOSURE: The skin is closed using a clear cyanoacrylic surgical adhesive (Figure CS6-4). No external sutures are required or recommended.

POST-OP EVALUATION: The patient should not lick or chew at the area.

FOLLOW-UP: The patient is re-evaluated at seven to ten days to assure adequate healing of the skin incision and that there is no swelling of the scrotum or discomfort.

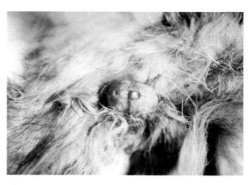

Figure CS6-1

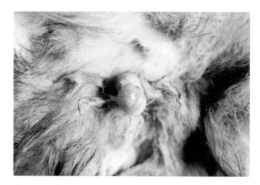

Figure CS6-2

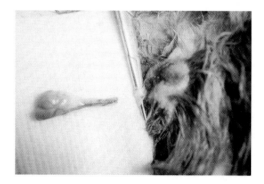

Figure CS6-3

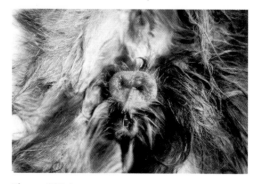

Figure CS6-4

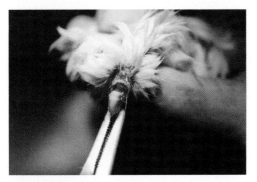

Figure CS7a-1

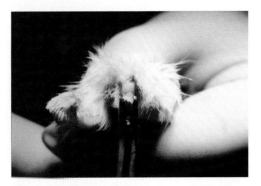

Figure CS7a-2

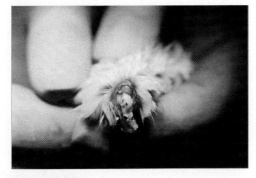

Figure CS7a-3

Figure CS7a-4

Case Study 7a
Feline Onychectomy

6-month-old male Domestic Shorthair, presented for laser onychectomy.

PROCEDURE: Dorsal approach to P2-P3 inter-phalangeal space, minimizing incision diameter to 4 mm to 5 mm and maximizing CO_2 laser's vaporization and cauterization abilities in the intra-articular space.

ANESTHESIA: Pre-medicated with medetomedine, butorphanol, and glycopyrrolate. Mask induction with isoflurane in oxygen. Maintenance of general anesthesia via endotracheal tube.

EQUIPMENT: 20-Watt CO_2 Novapulse™ laser with straight handpiece and 0.4 mm diameter metal or gold tip.

LASER SETTINGS:
Spot Diameter: 0.4 mm
Power Output: 4 W
Beam Output: CWSP or CWNSP, depending on comfort level and personal preference

TECHNIQUE: All fore toes are aseptically prepared with a chlorhexidine solution, and a 0.9% NaCl flush is applied as a final wetting agent to push back hair and allow good visualization of the dorsal interdigital space. No tourniquet is required or recommended. Each nail is individually grasped using 10 inch Mayo-Hegar needle holder just proximal to the ungual crest. A dorsal incision is made using the CO_2 laser in CW mode over the distal interphalangeal space (Figure CS7a-1). Avoid making a complete circumferential incision. Working through this dorsal incision, transect the dorsal annular ligament (Figure CS7a-2) and medial and lateral collateral distal interphalangeal ligaments. Next, identify and incise the dorsal aspect of the interphalangeal joint capsule (Figure CS7a-3). Once this is completed, apply light downward tension on the nail to expose the palmar interphalangeal joint capsule (Figure CS7a-3). Incise this using the CO_2 laser in CW mode. Once incised, the deep digital flexor tendon should become apparent at its insertion on the flexor process of P3. Direct the CO_2 laser energy toward the flexor process of P3 as you transect the deep digital flexor tendon (Figure CS7a-4). Once this is completed any small tissue tags remaining can be transected and P3 with the nail removed. The incision should be no larger than 4 mm to 5mm in diameter.

COMMENTS: Patient recovery should be uneventful. It is important to avoid dissociative drugs because they can lead to excitability, rough anesthetic recovery, hyperesthesia, and self-induced trauma to the incision sites. Patient may be discharged the same day of the procedure and sent home with shredded newspaper or wheat husk litter. Activity must be strictly reduced.

CLOSURE: Clear cyanoacrylic tissue adhesive on incision edges. No bandages are needed or recommended.

POST-OP EVALUATION: Patient should be able to bear weight before release from hospital.

FOLLOW UP: Recheck incisions and feet in ten to fourteen days.

Case Study 7b
Feline Onychectomy

6-month-old Domestic Shorthair cat, presented for laser onychectomy.

PROCEDURE: CO_2 laser-assisted onychectomy

ANESTHESIA: Pre-medicated with buprenorphine, acepromazine, and atropine. Mask induction with sevoflurane in oxygen. Maintenance of general anesthesia using isoflurane in oxygen via endotracheal tube.

EQUIPMENT: 20-Watt CO_2 Novapulse™ laser with straight handpiece. Oschner-type forceps.

LASER SETTINGS:
  Spot Diameter: 0.4 mm (small patients) or 0.8 mm (large patients)
  Power Output: 6 to 12 W
  Beam Output: CW

TECHNIQUE: All toes are cleansed, then rinsed with water, and a tourniquet may be placed above the elbow. Oschner forceps are used to clamp P3 just proximal to the ungual crest, and a single laser pass is made over the skin to free it from the joint capsule. (Figure CS7b-1). The laser transects the dorsal elastic ligament and the lateral (Figure CS7b-2) and medial (Figure CS7b-3) collateral distal interphalangeal ligaments, then finally the deep digital flexor tendon from their attachments on P3 (Figure CS7b-4). Any char on the skin incision is gently wiped away with sterile moistened gauze, then dried with sterile gauze. Finally, a small amount of surgical adhesive is applied to the skin edges only, then sealed closed. It is preferable to shape the toe to a natural and pleasing appearance (Figure CS7b-5).

COMMENTS: The patient should recover slowly and gradually from anesthesia. Rapid recovery may cause traumatic hemorrhage at the surgical site. An injectable broad-spectrum antibiotic is administered, and the patient is sent home with shredded newspaper to use as litterbox filler.

CLOSURE: 4-0 monofilament absorbable suture or surgical adhesive may be used to keep the socket closed during healing.

POST-OP EVALUATION: The patient should be walking comfortably immediately following anesthetic recovery.

FOLLOW-UP: None.

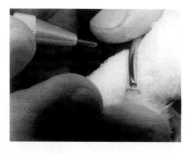

Figure CS7b-1

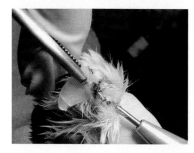

Figure CS7b-2

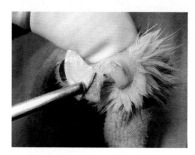

Figure CS7b-3

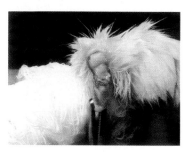

Figure CS7b-4

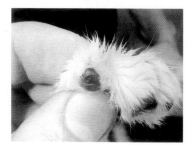

Figure CS7b-5

Case Study 8
Canine Digit Amputation

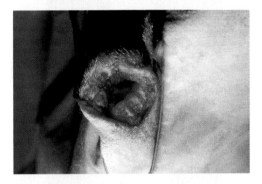

Figure CS8-1

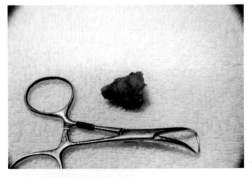

Figure CS8-2

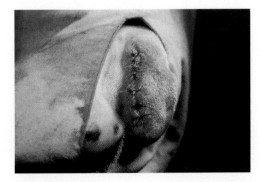

Figure CS8-3

Figure CS8-4

8-year-old male neutered Great Dane, presented for chronic infection and osteomyelitis of P3 of right forelimb digit 2.

PROCEDURE: Amputation of P3 of right forelimb digit 2.

ANESTHESIA: Pre-medicated with medetomedine, butorphanol, and glycopyrrolate. Mask induction with isoflurane in oxygen. Maintenance of general anesthesia via endotracheal tube.

EQUIPMENT: 20-Watt CO_2 Novapulse™ laser with straight handpiece and 0.4 mm diameter ceramic or gold tip.

LASER SETTINGS:
   Spot Diameter: 0.4 mm
   Power Output: 10 W
   Beam Output: CWSP skin incision, CWNSP dissection/dis-articulation

TECHNIQUE: A tourniquet is placed just prior to incising the skin. The digital pad should be preserved during this distal amputation. A transverse skin incision is made at the base of the nail and completely encircles the toe (Figure CS8-1). The articular surface of the distal second phalanx is maintained and charring should be avoided (Figure CS8-2). Incising the extensor and flexor tendons and the collateral ligaments disarticulates the joint as P3 is removed (Figure CS8-3). Defocusing the CO_2 laser beam to cause coagulation of the culprit vessel controls any small capillary bleeding. Alternatively, the identified vessel may be ligated using absorbable monofilament suture material.

COMMENTS: A bandage should be applied in this case due to the size of the incision and potential need for some pressure on the wound for the first twenty-four to forty-eight hours. The patient's recovery should be uneventful. It is important to avoid dissociative drugs because they can lead to excitability, rough anesthetic recovery, hyperesthesia, and self-induced trauma to the incision site. The patient is discharged the same day of the procedure. Restricted activity is recommended for one to two weeks.

CLOSURE: Simple interrupted monofilament absorbable suture material is used to reduce dead space. Skin is closed using non-absorbable monofilament in a simple interrupted pattern (Figure CS8-4). A pressure bandage is recommended but not required.

POST-OP EVALUATION: Patient should be able to bear weight upon recovery and release from hospital. Evaluate post-operative pain and provide appropriate pain medication. Broad-spectrum antibiotics should be administered until the sutures are removed.

FOLLOW-UP: Bandage removal and recheck of incision should be done at forty-eight hours. Suture removal at seven to ten days.

Case Study 9
Canine Dewclaw Amputation

1-year-old female spayed Labrador Retriever, presented for removal of forelimb dewclaws.

PROCEDURE: Amputation of first digit of both forelimbs.

ANESTHESIA: Pre-medicated with medetomedine, butorphanol, and glycopyrrolate. Mask induction with isoflurane in oxygen. Maintenance of general anesthesia via endotracheal tube.

EQUIPMENT: 20-Watt CO_2 Novapulse™ laser with straight handpiece and 0.4 mm diameter ceramic or gold tip.

LASER SETTINGS:
Spot Diameter: 0.4 mm
Power Output: 8 to 10 W
Beam Output: CWSP skin incision, CWNSP dissection/disarticulation

TECHNIQUE: A tourniquet is placed just prior to incising the skin. The digital pad should be included in the incision, because this will be removed to improve cosmetic appearance. A transverse elliptical skin incision is made around the nail base and includes the digital pad (Figure CS9-1). The dewclaw is then dissected free from underlying fascia and P3 and P2 are identified. The distal interphalangeal joint is identified and the joint disarticulated by incising the extensor and flexor tendons and the collateral ligaments (Figure CS9-2). The digit is removed (Figure CS9-3). The digital arteries and veins are ligated or cauterized depending on their respective sizes. The remainder of the joint capsule is identified and closed (Figure CS9-4).

COMMENTS: It is important to achieve a smooth surface for cosmetic effect. In some cases the metacarpal-phalangeal joint must be incised to provide adequate cosmetic effect. The CO_2 laser is preferred due to the small scar that remains after healing has taken place.

CLOSURE: Using simple interrupted monofilament absorbable suture to appose the subcutaneous tissues reduces dead space. Skin sutures are placed using simple interrupted monofilament non-absorbable material. A clear cyanoacrylic tissue adhesive is applied to the incision edges to further reduce post-operative scar formation. A light bandage wrap is applied for twenty-four to forty-eight hours.

POST-OP EVALUATION: Patient should be able to bear weight upon recovery and release from hospital. Owner should be instructed to not allow any licking or chewing of the surgical site.

FOLLOW UP: Bandage removal and recheck of incision should be done at forty-eight hours. Suture removal may be done at seven to ten days.

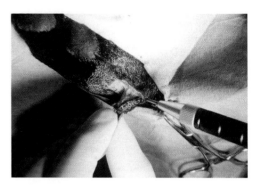
Figure CS9-1

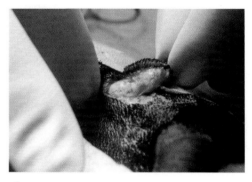
Figure CS9-2

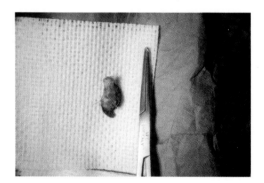
Figure CS9-3

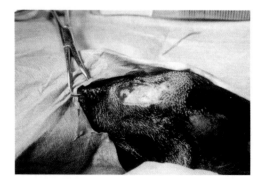
Figure CS9-4

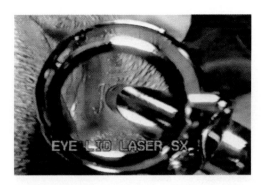

Figure CS10-1

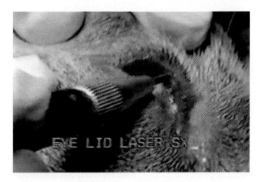

Figure CS10-2

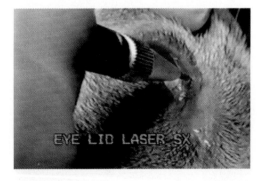

Figure CS10-3

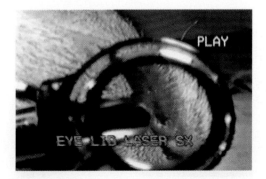

Figure CS10-4

Case Study 10
Distichia/Ectopic Cilia Ablation

2-year-old male neutered Weimerainer, presented for corneal edema associated with distichiasis/ectopic cilia.

PROCEDURE: Vaporization of cilia and its associated tarsal gland duct (Figure CS10-1).

ANESTHESIA: Pre-medicated with medetomedine, butorphanol, and glycopyrrolate. Mask induction with isoflurane in oxygen. Maintenance of general anesthesia via endotracheal tube. Prior to recovery, the cornea and lid margin of the eye should be treated with 1% proparacaine to further reduce discomfort.

EQUIPMENT: Magnifying scope, 20-Watt CO_2 Novapulse™ laser with straight handpiece and 0.3 mm metal tip.

LASER SETTINGS:
    Spot Diameter: 0.3 mm
    Power Output: 3-5 W
    Beam Output: Single pulse 200-500 msec, superpulse

TECHNIQUE: The atypical cilia are identified using a magnifying scope. The lumen of a 0.3 mm tip is guided over the cilia. The tip should be 0.25mm to 0.5 mm from the surface of conjunctiva or eyelid margin and directed over the associated tarsal gland (Figure CS10-2). CO_2 laser energy is delivered in a single pulse output setting for 200 msec SP for small ectopic cilia and for 500 msec SP or larger distichia. Two to four pulses will be needed to vaporize the cilia and the associated tarsal gland (Figure CS10-3). Upon vaporization of the tarsal gland a small amount of gray debris will be noted at the laser trough site. This indicates that the tarsal gland has been vaporized and the cilia will most likely not grow back.

COMMENTS: If char is noted during the pulsing process, it should be lavaged away using sterile 0.9% NaCl. Care must be taken not to touch the laser tip to the corneal surface. Pulse until you are confident that the tarsal gland has been effectively vaporized. Some tissue contracture immediately adjacent to the laser trough will be noted if the power density is too low.

CLOSURE: No sutures or other form of closure is needed. The laser troughs will granulate within four to five days without scarring or disfigurement (Figure CS10-4).

POST-OP EVALUATION: Treated area and the cornea should be evaluated to ensure proper healing and resolution of clinical symptoms, e.g., corneal edema, epiphora.

FOLLOW-UP: Treated area should be re-evaluated in twelve weeks to ensure that cilia has not regrown.

Case Study 11
Elongated Soft Palate Resection

5-year-old male American Bulldog, presented for surgical sterilization and history of snoring.

PROCEDURE: Excision of redundant and excessive uvular tissue obstructing the laryngeal airway.

ANESTHESIA: Pre-medicate with buprenorphine, acepromazine, glycopyrrolate, and oxygen mask. Induce anesthesia with intravenous propofol. An endotracheal tube may be placed for highest safety, but may interfere with the procedure in some cases. Anesthesia may be maintained with slow propofol infusion to effect, or inhalant anesthetic.

EQUIPMENT: 20-Watt CO_2 Novapulse™ laser, backstopped handpiece, forceps or stay suture for traction.

LASER SETTINGS:
    Spot Diameter: 0.8 mm
    Power Output: 10 to 15 W
    Beam Output: CW

TECHNIQUE: Traction is placed upon the distal midline of the elongated soft palate (Figure CS11-1). The surgeon makes a visual estimation of the amount of tissue to remove. Begin at the lateral margin of the palate and vaporize tissue in a straight path heading to the opposite side (Figure CS11-2).

COMMENTS: The goal is for the new soft palate to conform to the shape of the epiglottis and just barely make contact with it (Figure CS11-3). Most dogs will enjoy free breathing immediately with reduced stridor. Some dogs may have increased breath sounds due to the increased flow of air through the oropharynx, which is the most desirable outcome of this procedure.

CLOSURE: None required. It is contraindicated to wipe char since this may cause oropharyngeal bleeding. A single dose of a broad-spectrum antibiotic is administered.

POST-OP EVALUATION: There should be a noticeable decrease in respiratory effort and stridor following the procedure.

FOLLOW-UP: None

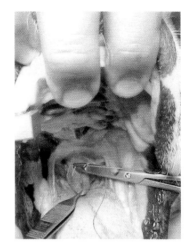

Figure CS11-1

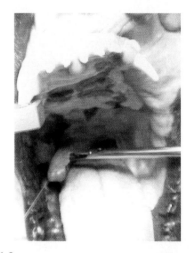

Figure CS11-2

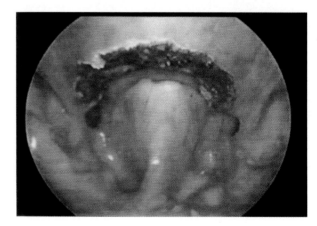

Figure CS11-3

Case Study 12
Feline Ovariohysterectomy

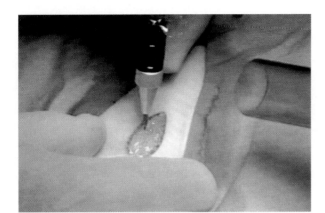

Figure CS12-1

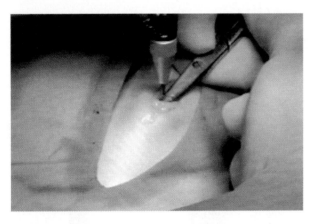

Figure CS12-2

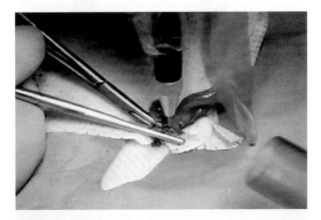

Figure CS12-3

6-month-old female Domestic Shorthair, presented for CO_2 laser-assisted ovariohysterectomy.

PROCEDURE: Incision, laparotomy, hemostasis, and removal of reproductive tract.

ANESTHESIA: Pre-medicated with medetomedine, butorphanol, and glycopyrrolate. Mask induction with isoflurane in oxygen. Maintenance of general anesthesia via endotracheal tube.

EQUIPMENT: 20-Watt CO_2 Novapulse™ laser with straight handpiece and 0.4 mm ceramic, metal, or gold tip.

LASER SETTINGS:
  Spot Diameter: 0.4 mm
  Power Output: 8 to 10 W
  Beam Output: SP skin/abdominal incision,
  CW transection of uterine horns, body, and broad ligament

TECHNIQUE: Laser handpiece is held perpendicular to the skin at a position halfway between the umbilicus and the pubis along the ventral midline (Figure CS12-1). The skin is tensed and a single-pass, full-thickness laser trough is produced using SP. Fatty tissue is undermined using straight Metzenbaum scissors. The linea alba is identified and Adson tissue forceps are used to tent it up. The laser handpiece is directed at a 45-degree angle to the linea and a laser stab incision is made into the linea using SP. Metzenbaum scissors are then advanced into the stab incision and the linea lifted slightly to provide tension and backstop protection. The laser handpiece is again directed perpendicular to the linea and a single pass is made, CW, to produce an abdominal incision (Figure CS12-2). All char is wiped away before proceeding to remove the reproductive tract.

The right or left uterine horn is located and exteriorized by the use of an ovariohysterectomy hook. The ovary is identified and lifted out of the incision. The suspensory ligament is stretched and transected using the CO_2 laser CW. The ovarian pedicle is double-clamped. Absorbable monofilament sutures are used as ligatures. A wetted 0.9% NaCl gauze is placed as a backstop under the pedicle. The laser handpiece is directed perpendicular, and targeted between the edges of the clamps. The uterine horn is transected proximal to the ovarian pedicle (Figure CS12-3). The pedicle is observed for any bleeding, then allowed to slide back into the abdominal cavity. The procedure is repeated on the opposite side.

The broad ligament is identified from both uterine horns and placed over a wetted 0.9% NaCl gauze. The laser handpiece is directed perpendicular to the ligament (Figure CS12-4). The broad ligament is then divided using CW, then observed for any bleeding or leakage from vessels running through it. The uterine body is exteriorized and its vessels identified. Two clamps are placed on the uterine body cranial to the cervix. The uterine arteries are individually ligated proximal to the most proximal clamp. The laser handpiece is again directed perpendicular between the two clamps. The body is transected (Figure CS12-5) between the two clamps. The uterine horn is mass ligated proximal to the most proximal clamp. The clamp is removed and the pedicle is inspected for bleeding. The pedicle is allowed to fall back into the abdomen. The abdomen is examined for evidence of any bleeding.

COMMENTS: The use of a CO_2 laser for transection of various structures and ligaments reduces hemorrhage, which is reported as the most common cause of death after ovariohysterectomy.

CLOSURE: Routine closure of the linea alba, subcuticular tissues, and skin is completed. Make sure that no char is present on the skin incision edges before suturing. A gel to enhance healing (Facilitator™) may be applied to the incision to protect the incision and speed the healing rate.

POST-OP EVALUATION: Patient should be comfortable and fully mobile at time of discharge. Owners should be instructed to reduce pet's activity for five to seven days. Patients often have significantly reduced pain following anesthetic recovery, therefore they return to normal activity much more rapidly than those undergoing conventional surgery.

FOLLOW-UP: A recheck and suture removal in ten to fourteen days is recommended. If used, skin sutures should be removed at this time.

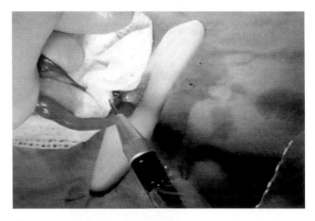

Figure CS12-4

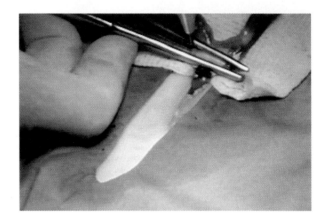

Figure CS12-5

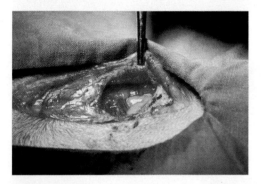

Figure CS13-1

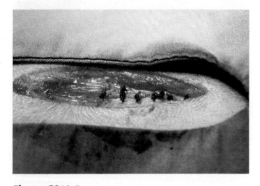

Figure CS13-2

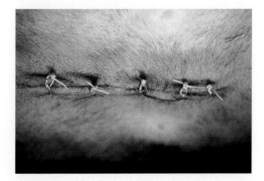

Figure CS13-3

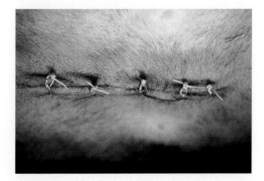

Figure CS13-4

Case Study 13
Umbilical Hernia Repair

6-month-old female spayed Golden Retriever, presented for ovariohysterectomy and umbilical herniorrhapy.

PROCEDURE: Repair and closure of uncomplicated congenital umbilical hernia.

ANESTHESIA: Pre-medicated with medetomedine, butorphanol, and glycopyrrolate. Mask induction with isoflurane in oxygen. Maintenance of general anesthesia via endotracheal tube.

EQUIPMENT: 20-Watt CO_2 Novapulse™ laser with straight handpiece and 0.4 mm metal or gold tip.

LASER SETTINGS:
  Spot Diameter: 0.4 mm
  Power Output: 8 to 10 W
  Beam Output: SP skin incision, abdominal muscle incision, CW resection of herniated omentum or falciform ligament

TECHNIQUE: When an umbilical hernia is corrected at the time of ovariohysterectomy, the incision can be extended to the hernia, or an elliptical incision is made around the base of the large sac to remove redundant skin tissue (Figure CS13-1). The herniated sac is identified and dissected free from associated fat and fascia. The sac is then lifted up and an elliptical incision is made through the abdominal musculature in CW. Immediately adjacent to the sac, the sac is lifted up from the surrounding tissue and turned over to evaluate the herniated material for any signs of entrapped small intestines or other organs. The omental tissue or falciform tissue is resected off of the muscle/ring pedicle. The pedicle is removed and the abdominal tissue allowed to slide back into the abdomen (Figure CS13-2).

COMMENTS: Removal of char is important from both the muscular incision and the skin incision. This technique allows for more rapid access to the hernia for evaluation of potential entrapped tissue. Muscle incised with a CO_2 laser bleeds less and produces less post-operative pain.

CLOSURE: Simple interrupted monofilament absorbable suture is used to close the fresh muscle edges (Figure CS13-3). Skin is closed in a routine simple interrupted pattern using non-absorbable monofilament suture material (Figure CS13-4).

POST-OP EVALUATION: Resolution of hernia should be complete. Wound edges should be well apposed with no evidence of tension on the incision site.

FOLLOW-UP: Abdominal incision should be re-evaluated in ten to fourteen days. Suture removal is generally done at this time.

Case Study 14a
Canine Lower Eyelid Entropion Repair

10-year-old male neutered Cocker Spaniel, presented for surgical repair of bilateral lower eyelid entropion: 180 degree roll-in of lid margins from normal position (Figure CS14a-1).

PROCEDURE: Contracture of collagen within the deep tissues of the lower eyelid margins. This facilitates roll-out of lid margins to a normal anatomical position.

ANESTHESIA: Pre-medicated with medetomedine, butorphanol, and glycopyrrolate. Mask induction with isoflurane in oxygen. Maintenance of general anesthesia via endotracheal tube.

EQUIPMENT: 20-Watt CO_2 Novapulse™ laser with straight handpiece and 0.8 mm ceramic tip.

LASER SETTINGS:
   Spot Diameter: 0.8 mm
   Power Output: 3 to 4 W
   Beam Output: CW

TECHNIQUE: After aseptic surgical preparation of the lower eyelid margin, including removal of overlying hair, the handpiece is placed perpendicular to the eyelid margin. Laser energy is introduced to the eyelid margin tissue in the form of "X" striations in a linear pattern. Each "X" is approximately 3 mm to 4 mm and 1 mm to 2 mm apart (Figure CS14a-2). The laser tip should be placed at such a distance above the skin that maximal contracture is noted upon laser/tissue interaction. The "X" pattern will create a circular contraction zone, everting the eyelid margin corresponding to each "X." It is important not to create full-thickness incisions with the "X" pattern, because this will cause release of the tissue and relaxation of the contracted area. If a single row of "X"s does not provide complete resolution of the affected eyelid margin, a second row of "X"s can be produced below the first row and in the same fashion (Figure CS14a-3). In the majority of cases this should be sufficient to provide for return to normal anatomic position of the eyelid margin (Figure CS14a-4).

COMMENTS: If the surgeon has access to a mechanical pattern scanner, a single line of laser energy can be scanned over the same area as would be under the "X"s. The same power output and beam output can be used. A second scanned line can be applied to the area of the second row of "X"s. The advantage we have noted is a more uniform contracture of tissue and improved roll-out of the affected eyelid margin. A second treatment, performed at a later date, is sometimes required in young dogs or severe cases.

CLOSURE: The treated area is gently cleaned with sterile 0.9% NaCl-soaked gauze sponges to remove char. A topical antibiotic cream can be applied to the area for seven to ten days.

POST-OP EVALUATION: The area should have minimal swelling. Normal anatomical position of the eyelid margin should be present upon anesthetic recovery.

FOLLOW-UP: Patient should be rechecked in seven to fourteen days and any mild scabs lifted off the site. Normal hair re-growth should begin to be noted.

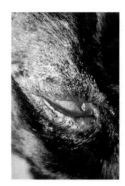

Figure CS14a-1

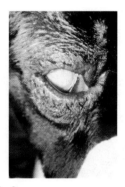

Figure CS14a-2

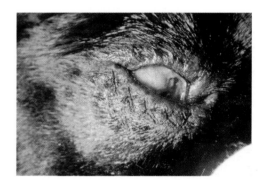

Figure CS14a-3

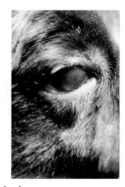

Figure CS14a-4

Case Study 14b
Canine Lower Eyelid Entropion Repair

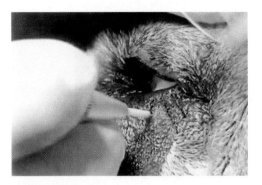

Figure CS14b-1

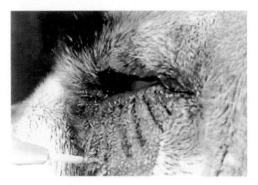

Figure CS14b-2

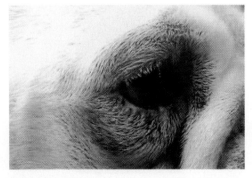

Figure CS14b-3

Figure CS14b-4

6-year-old female spayed Old English Bulldog presented for surgical repair of bilateral lower eyelid entropion: 180 degree roll-in of lid margins from normal position (Figure CS14b-1).

PROCEDURE: Contracture of collagen deep within the dermis of the lower eyelids to facilitate roll-out of lid margins to normal anatomical position.

ANESTHESIA: Pre-medicated with medetomedine, butorphanol, and glycopyrrolate. Mask induction with isoflurane in oxygen. Maintenance of general anesthesia via endotracheal tube.

EQUIPMENT: 20-Watt CO_2 Novapulse™ laser with straight handpiece and 0.8 mm ceramic tip.

LASER SETTINGS:
Spot Diameter: 0.8 mm
Power Output: 8 to 10 W
Beam Output: SP

TECHNIQUE: The cornea of each eye is protected with water-soluble medical lubricating jelly (K-Y Jelly™). A single well-placed pass with a hair clipper is used to prepare the skin. After this, the lower eyelid is cleansed very gently, using sterile saline, to remove any hair or stubble. The handpiece is targeted perpendicular to the lateral eyelid margin (Figure CS14b-2). The laser tip should produce a focused beam at a distance above the skin that causes maximal effect. Laser energy is introduced to the eyelid margin tissue in the form of radiating streaks in a linear pattern away from the margin. Working lateral to medial, each subsequent pass is approximately 1 mm to 2 mm apart and as lengthy as needed to cause eversion of the lower lid. In the majority of cases this should be sufficient to provide for return to normal anatomic position of the eyelid margin (Figure CS14b-3).

COMMENTS: This desirable effect causes the skin to tighten and shorten along the longitudinal axis of the laser beam pass. This effect is immediately visible to the surgeon and "what you see is what you get" as far the degree of change created. The pass should continue as long as the effect is noticed. When the effect stops, the surgeon should stop lasing and move on to another area. If unsatisfactory changes have occurred with one pass, it is NOT advisable to make a second pass over the first. A second treatment is sometimes required in young dogs or severe cases.

CLOSURE: The surgical area is gently cleaned with sterile 0.9% NaCl-soaked gauze sponges to gently remove char. Avoid aggressive wiping because this effect may stretch the tissues and nullify any produced surgical contracture. We recommend a gentle cool compress for three days following the procedure, and an Elizabethan collar.

POST-OP EVALUATION: The area should have minimal swelling. Normal anatomical position of the eyelid margin should be present upon anesthetic recovery.

FOLLOW-UP: Patient should be rechecked at both seven and twenty-one days. Normal hair re-growth should begin to be noted. Mild scarring may occur. Any blepharospasm, epiphora, or corneal edema should all be resolved (Figure CS14b-4).

Case Study 15a
Canine Aural Hematoma

5-year-old male neutered Golden Retriever, presented for surgical repair of an aural hematoma of the right pinna (Figure CS15a-1).

PROCEDURE: Creation of incisional drainage holes on the medial surface of the pinna. Stay sutures are placed to eliminate dead space and facilitate re-adherence of auricular cartilage to skin.

ANESTHESIA: Pre-medicated with medetomedine, butorphanol, and glycopyrrolate. Mask induction with isoflurane in oxygen. Maintenance of general anesthesia via endotracheal tube.

EQUIPMENT: 20-Watt CO_2 Novapulse™ laser with straight handpiece and 0.4 mm metal or gold tip.

LASER SETTINGS:
   Spot Diameter: 0.4 mm
   Power Output: 8 to 10 W
   Beam Output: SP

TECHNIQUE: The ear is prepared for sterile surgery. All hair is clipped away from the medial surface of the pinna. The laser handpiece is directed perpendicular to the skin surface at the appropriate focal distance (Figure CS15a-2). Drainage holes are created equidistant from each other sufficient to allow for adequate drainage of the hematoma. Clotted blood and fibrin are removed using tissue forceps (Figure CS15a-3). Stay sutures are then placed through the pinna, incorporating both medial and lateral layers of cartillage and skin, thus securing a reduction in dead space (Figure CS15a-4).

COMMENTS: The number of drainage holes and stay sutures must be sufficient to eliminate any dead space and allow for adequate continuous drainage during healing.

CLOSURE: We use a light pressure wrap that is sutured in place at the base of the pinna and allowed to remain in place for three to seven days. The individual surgeon must decide on the appropriate amount of bandaging material that is needed to absorb the drainage.

POST-OP EVALUATION: The pinna wrap is removed in three to seven days and the client is given written discharge instructions pertaining to home maintenance and care.

FOLLOW-UP: Sutures should be re-evaluated in fourteen days and the drainage holes checked for patency. If no drainage is noted and/or drainage holes have healed, the sutures can be removed. The pinna should return to normal anatomical position and thickness. Scars should be minimal and hair re-growth uneventful (Figure CS15a-5).

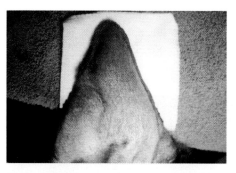

Figure CS15a-1

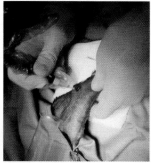

Figure CS15a-2

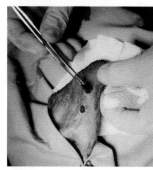

Figure CS15a-3

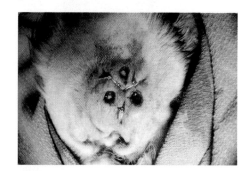

Figure CS15a-4

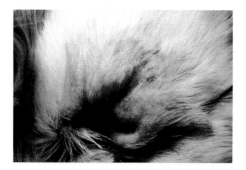

Figure CS15a-5

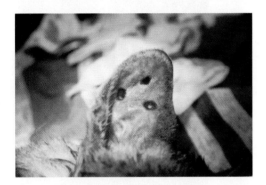

Figure CS15b-1

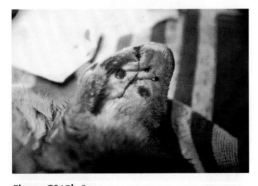

Figure CS15b-2

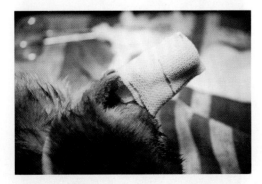

Figure CS15b-3

Case Study 15b
Feline Aural Hematoma

7-year-old male neutered Domestic Shorthair, presented for surgical repair of an aural hematoma (Figure CS15b-1).

PROCEDURE: Creation of incisional drainage holes on the medial surface of the pinna. Stay sutures are placed to eliminate dead space and facilitate re-adherence of auricular cartilage to skin.

ANESTHESIA: Pre-medicated with medetomedine, butorphanol, and glycopyrrolate. Mask induction with isoflurane in oxygen. Maintenance of general anesthesia via endotracheal tube.

EQUIPMENT: 20-Watt CO_2 Novapulse™ laser with straight handpiece and 0.4 mm metal or gold tip.

LASER SETTINGS:
  Spot Diameter: 0.4 mm
  Power Output: 6 to 8 W
  Beam Output: CW

TECHNIQUE: The ear is prepared for sterile surgery. All hair is clipped away from the medial surface. The laser handpiece is placed perpendicular to the skin surface at appropriate focal distance. Drainage holes are created equidistant from each other sufficient to allow for adequate drainage of the hematoma. Clotted blood and fibrin are removed using tissue forceps (Figure CS15b-2). Stay sutures are then placed through the pinna, incorporating both medial and lateral layers of cartilage and skin, thus securing a reduction in dead space (Figure CS15b-3).

COMMENTS: The number of drainage holes and stay sutures must be sufficient to eliminate any dead space and allow for adequate continuous drainage during healing.

CLOSURE: We use a light pressure wrap that is sutured in place at the base of the pinna and allowed to remain in place for three to seven days. The individual surgeon must decide on the appropriate amount of bandaging material needed to absorb the drainage (Figure CS15b-4).

POST-OP EVALUATION: The pinna wrap is removed in three to seven days and the client is given written discharge instructions pertaining to home maintenance and care.

FOLLOW-UP: Sutures should be re-evaluated in fourteen days and the drainage holes checked for patency. If no drainage is noted and/or drainage holes have healed, the sutures can be removed. The pinna should return to normal anatomical position and thickness. Scars should be minimal and hair re-growth uneventful.

Figure CS15b-4

Case Study 16a
Uncomplicated Acral Lick Granuloma

7-year-old male neutered Bichon-Frise, presented for evaluation of chronic acral lick granuloma of the right foreleg (Figure CS16a-1). Treatment options include using CO_2 laser energy.

PROCEDURE: Ablation/vaporization of granulation tissue overlying normal dermis.

ANESTHESIA: Pre-medicated with hydromorphone sedative/analgesic. Local ring block using 2% mepivicaine infusion.

EQUIPMENT: 20-Watt CO_2 Novapulse™ laser with straight handpiece and 1.4 mm metal tip.

LASER SETTINGS:
Spot Diameter: 1.4 mm
Power Output: 15 to 20 W
Beam Output: 20 Hz at 50 msec SP

TECHNIQUE: The area to be treated is cleaned of debris and crusted material. The CO_2 laser is applied to remove the overlying granulation tissue at the affected area. The granulation tissue should be removed down to or slightly below the adjoining normal epidermal and dermal layers. The treated area should be flushed to remove any char buildup after each pass with the laser. Upon completion, any remaining char (Figure CS16a-2) should be aggressively cleaned from the surface.

COMMENTS: In our experience, a significant number of these cases have underlying metabolic, orthopedic, or behavioral issues that have led to this condition. It is always advisable for the clinician to do a complete diagnostic evaluation of the patient, including laboratory blood values, T4, TSH, Cortisol values, radiographs of the affected limb, culture/sensitivity of the affected area, and biopsy of a section of abnormal tissue with adjoining normal dermis.

CLOSURE: The treated area can be covered with a wound-management dressing for twenty-four to forty-eight hours. Re-evaluation at that time is recommended. A topical antibiotic cream can then be dispensed for application at home. If treated aggressively, resolution of the abnormal tissue can be completed in one treatment. A relatively cosmetic appearance should be the expected therapeutic outcome with some hair re-growth considered optimal (Figure CS16a-3).

POST-OP EVALUATION: The area should be evaluated every two weeks for a six-week period to ensure complete healing. If there is evidence of recurrence the diagnostic work-up should be re-evaluated for other possible origins of the acral lick granuloma. Re-treatment of the area can be completed as before.

FOLLOW-UP: Annual follow-up should be conducted during any physical examination.

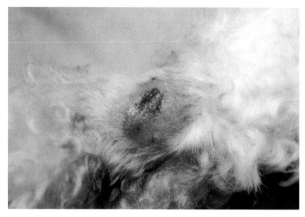

Figure CS16a-1

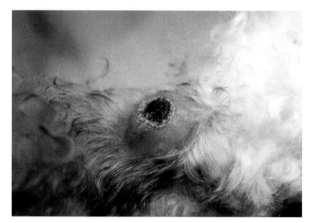

Figure CS16a-2

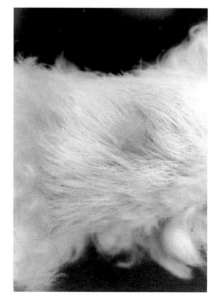

Figure CS16a-3

Case Study 16b
Multi-Factoral Acral Lick Granuloma

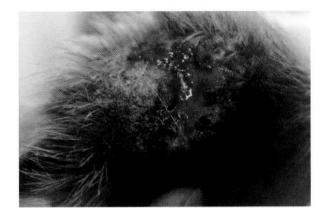

Figure CS16b-1

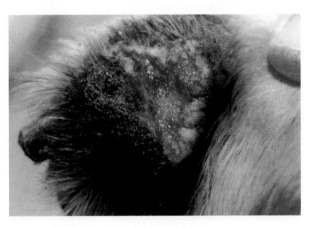

Figure CS16b-2

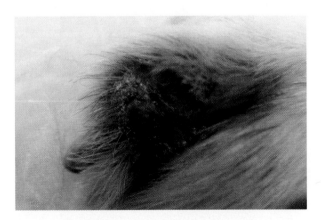

Figure CS16b-3

3-year-old male neutered English Mastiff, presented for surgical removal of a severe acral lick granuloma overlying the third digit of the right forelimb (Figure CS16b-1).

PROCEDURE: Resection and de-bulking of excessive granulation tissue using CO_2 laser energy. This is followed by ablation/vaporization of remaining granulation tissue overlying the normal dermis.

ANESTHESIA: Pre-medicated with medetomedine, butorphanol, and glycopyrrolate. Mask induction with isoflurane in oxygen. Maintenance of general anesthesia via endotracheal tube.

EQUIPMENT: 20-Watt CO_2 Novapulse™ laser with straight handpiece and 0.4 mm ceramic tip for resection. Mechanical scanner with 3 mm pattern scans for ablation/vaporization of remaining granulation tissue.

LASER SETTINGS:
Resection work
    Spot Diameter: 0.4 mm
    Power Output: 10 to 15 W
    Beam Output: SP
Ablative/Vaporization work
    Spot Diameter: 3 mm pattern scan using a 0.8 mm daisywheel
      spot
    Power Output: 10 W
    Beam Output: SP

TECHNIQUE: The region with the acral lick granuloma is evaluated and aseptically prepared. The bulk of the overlying granulation tissue is resected in a wedge or broad surface resection. It is important not to produce a full-thickness resection down to the underlying fascia, ligament, tendon, or muscle structures. Once the majority of granulation tissue is removed, the area is flushed and the char removed. The scanner attachment is then set up for the ablation/vaporization of any remaining granulation tissue down to or slightly below the level of the surrounding normal dermis. For severe cases, multiple resurfacing may be needed for complete and cosmetic resolution.

COMMENTS: In our experience, a significant number of these cases have underlying metabolic, orthopedic, or behavioral issues that have led to this condition. It is always advisable for the clinician to do a complete diagnostic evaluation of the patient, including laboratory blood values, T4, TSH, cortisol values, radiographs of the affected limb, culture/sensitivity of the affected area, and biopsy of a section of abnormal tissue with adjoining normal dermis. In this case un-united anconeal processes were identified in the elbow joint.

CLOSURE: The treated area can be covered with a wound management dressing for twenty-four to forty-eight hours. Re-evaluation at that time is recommended. A topical antibiotic cream can then be dispensed for application at home. If treated aggressively, significant resolution of this abnormal tissue can be completed in one treatment (Figure CS16b-2). Multiple re-treatments using ablation/vaporization is sometimes required, such as in this case (Figure CS16b-3). A relatively cosmetic appearance should be the expected therapeutic outcome (Figure CS16b-4) with some hair re-growth considered optimal.

POST-OP EVALUATION: The area should be evaluated every two weeks for a six-week period to ensure complete healing. If there is evidence of recurrence the diagnostic work-up should be re-evaluated for other possible origins of the acral lick granuloma. Re-treatment of the area can be completed as before.

FOLLOW-UP: Annual follow-up should be conducted during any physical examination.

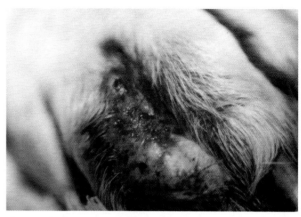

Figure CS16b-4

Case Study 17
Feline Fibrosarcoma Removal

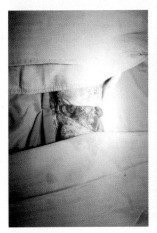

Figure CS17-1

Figure CS17-2   **Figure CS17-3**

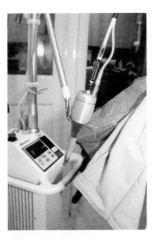

Figure CS17-4

7-year-old female spayed Domestic Shorthair presented for treatment of a vaccine-associated fibrosarcoma located in the subcutaneous layer and musculature of the right dorsal midline.

PROCEDURE: Use of CO_2 laser energy for wide margin incision and removal of neoplasm and surrounding tissue for histopathology to determine extent of soft tissue invasion.

ANESTHESIA: Pre-medicated with medetomedine, butorphanol, and glycopyrrolate. Mask induction with isoflurane in oxygen. Maintenance of general anesthesia via endotracheal tube.

EQUIPMENT: 20-Watt CO_2 Novapulse™ laser with straight handpiece and 0.4 mm metal or gold tip, mechanical scanner with 3 mm pattern scans.

LASER SETTINGS:
Skin incision and resection of tissue
    Spot Diameter: 0.4 mm
    Power Output: 8 to 10 W
    Beam Output: SP
Tumor bed ablation/vaporization
    Spot Diameter: 3 mm pattern scan using a 0.8 mm daisywheel
      spot
    Power Output: 10 W
    Beam Output: SP

TECHNIQUE: Surgical removal of the overlying dermis and primary mass (Figures CS17-1 and CS17-2) should be accomplished to allow for at least 2 cm of apparently normal tissue (Figure CS17-3). The fibrosarcoma mass should also be resected at least one additional muscle group deep to its origin. Excellent division of both skin and muscle tissue can be achieved with CO_2 laser energy. Good visualization is provided and wound margins can be more accurately inspected for any signs of gross tumor remaining. Once the surgeon is satisfied with the margin widths and excision of the tumor, a mechanical pattern scanner (Figure CS17-4) can be used to cause resurfacing by ablation/vaporization over the entire surgical region. We theorize that this can improve the potential for removal of any seed cells or fibroblast tendrils that may remain undetected. The area is then flushed and wiped aggressively to remove any char.

COMMENTS: After the initial excision has been completed, all drapes, instruments, and surgical supplies that have been in contact with the neoplastic tissue should be removed from the surgeon and patient. A new sterile surgical set up should be available and provided by the surgical technician. This also can minimize re-seeding the area with neoplastic cells from the original tumor.

CLOSURE: Standard reconstruction closure is recommended to reduce dead space and tension. Healing should provide for a cosmetic appearance in the future.

POST-OP EVALUATION: Suspected fibrosarcomas and all tumors of the skin should be submitted for histopathology. Once the diagnosis has been made, consultation with a veterinary oncologist is recommended for current treatment options.

FOLLOW-UP: The treated area should be re-examined once every four to six weeks for evidence of tumor recurrence. If re-identified early, repeated surgical treatments may be considered to increase the lifespan and quality of life of the patient.

Case Study 18
Canine Lateral Ear Canal Resection

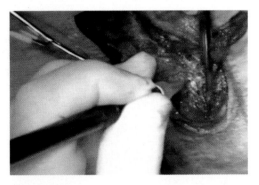

Figure CS18-1

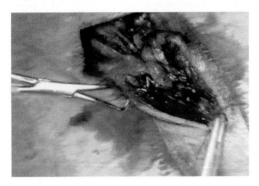

Figure CS18-2

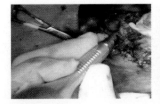

Figure CS18-3

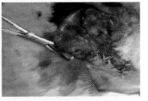

Figure CS18-4 **Figure CS18-5**

7-year-old male neutered Scottish Terrier, presented for lateral ear canal resection for management of chronic proliferative otitis externa.

PROCEDURE: Lacroix-Zepp technique of lateral external ear canal resection, using incisional and excisional CO_2 laser surgical proficiency. Any remaining hyperplastic inflammatory tissue may be ablated/vaporized using a mechanical scanner.

ANESTHESIA: Pre-medicated with medetomedine, butorphanol, and glycopyrrolate. Mask induction with isoflurane in oxygen. Maintenance of general anesthesia via endotracheal tube.

EQUIPMENT: 20-Watt CO_2 Novapulse™ laser with straight handpiece and 0.4 mm metal or gold tip, mechanical scanner with 3 mm pattern scans.

LASER SETTINGS:
Skin incision and resection of lateral ear canal
    Spot Diameter: 0.4 mm
    Power Output: 8 to 10 W
    Beam Output: SP
Granulation tissue bed ablation/vaporization
    Spot Diameter: 3 mm pattern scan using a 0.8 mm daisywheel spot
    Power Output: 10 W
    Beam Output: SP

TECHNIQUE: A standard Lacroix-Zepp technique is employed using the advantages of CO_2 laser energy for incision and excision. The ear canal is lavaged and the pinna and overlying skin prepared for surgery. Directing the handpiece perpendicular to the skin, a rostral and caudal margin skin incision is made over the vertical canal using 0.4 mm tip 8 to 10 W SP. The incisions are joined ventrally (Figure CS18-1). The skin flap is lifted up and used as a handle to apply tension to the subcutaneous tissue and vertical ear canal cartilage. The handpiece is then directed perpendicular to the lateral wall of the ear canal. Both a rostral and caudal margin incision is made through the lateral auricular cartilage to a ventral point just below the end of the vertical ear canal. A non-traumatic tissue clamp can be applied to the auricular cartilage to be used as a guide for laser energy delivery (Figure CS18-2). The proximal two-thirds of the auricular cartilage flap is excised. The remaining one-third is reflected downward and sutured ventrally to the edge of the ventral skin incision (Figure CS18-3). This creates a "drain board" of cartilage that can be sutured to the skin margins using monofilament non-absorbable suture. Once this is accomplished the scanner attachment can be used to ablate/vaporize hyperplastic inflammatory tissue down to the level of normal auricular cartilage on the medial wall of the vertical ear canal (Figure CS18-4). The area is flushed to remove char and irrigate the horizontal external ear canal.

COMMENTS: Typically, no bandaging is needed, because the drainage is minimal (Figure CS18-5).

POST-OP EVALUATION: The ear should be re-evaluated at both seven and fourteen days. Sutures can be removed at this time.

FOLLOW-UP: Topical and systemic antibiotics are indicated for fourteen days postoperatively.

Case Study 19
Ablation of Small Skin Mass

9-year-old female spayed Retriever, presented for removal of a small dermal adenoma on the right flank.

PROCEDURE: Outpatient ablation of surface mass using CO_2 laser energy.

ANESTHESIA: Local infusion of 2% lidocaine and 2% mepivicaine (50:50 mixture) ring block.

EQUIPMENT: 20-Watt CO_2 Novapulse™ laser with straight handpiece and 0.8 mm ceramic tip.

LASER SETTINGS:
   Spot Diameter: 0.8 mm
   Power Output: 12 to 15 W
   Beam Output: CW

TECHNIQUE: The area is aseptically prepared and shaved (Figure CS19-1). The area is then blocked locally with an infusion block. The surface of the mass is removed via surface excision by placing the tip parallel to the dermis and removing the mass. This is prepared in formalin for histopathology. Placing the tip perpendicular to the dermis and focusing the laser energy into the area of the mass ablates the remainder of the mass deep to the surface. After each pass the char should be removed to evaluate underlying tissue. The laser trough should be deepened until no evidence of atypical tissue is noted. Once the surgeon is satisfied with the mass ablation, the laser tip can be defocused and the wound edges lased. This will produce a contractile effect to the surface collagen of the surrounding dermis and contract the wound (Figure CS19-2). The effect is to reduce the total surface area of the defect by up to 50%.

COMMENTS: Masses that are less than 0.5 cm in diameter typically can be easily removed during regular examination visits. The temperament of both the patient and the client should be taken into account before considering doing this procedure during an office appointment.

CLOSURE: All char is cleaned away and the trough is treated with a wound management agent or topical antibiotic.

POST-OP EVALUATION: The area should be evaluated for patient comfort and hemostasis before release. A topical antibiotic should be dispensed. Mild analgesics may also be prescribed.

FOLLOW-UP: No follow-up is typically needed for this procedure. The wound will typically resolve to a small stelate scar in about two to three weeks.

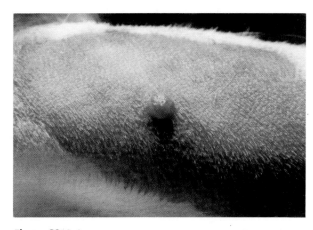

Figure CS19-1

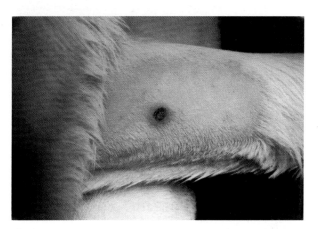

Figure CS19-2

Case Study 20
Removal of Canine Mast Cell Tumor

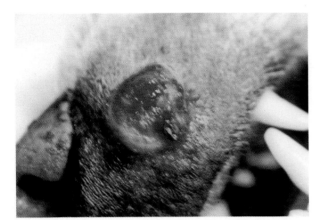

Figure CS20-1

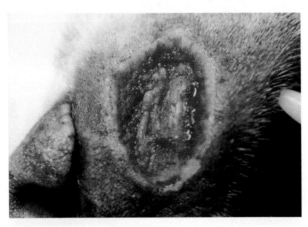

Figure CS20-2

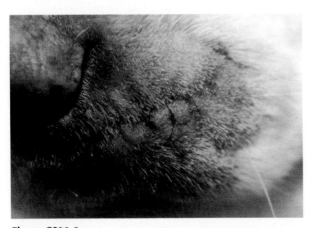

Figure CS20-3

6-year-old male neutered Labrador Retriever, presented for excision and ablation of mast cell tumor from the left rostral maxillary lip region.

PROCEDURE: This mast cell tumor was removed using a combination of excision and vaporization with CO_2 laser energy, providing good surgical margins and adequate retention of nerve and vascular supply to the rostral region of the lip in this patient.

ANESTHESIA: Pre-medicated with diphenhydramine, medetomedine, butorphanol, and glycopyrrolate. Mask induction with isoflurane in oxygen. Maintenance of general anesthesia via endotracheal tube.

EQUIPMENT: 20-Watt CO_2 Novapulse™ laser with straight handpiece and 0.4 mm metal or gold tip, mechanical scanner with 3 mm pattern scans.

LASER SETTINGS:
Resection of mass providing good margins
    Spot Diameter: 0.4 mm gold tip
    Power Output: 10 W
    Beam Output: SP
Vaporization of margins deep to surface
    Spot Diameter: 3 mm pattern scan using a 0.8 mm daisywheel spot
    Power Output: 10 W
    Beam Output: SP

TECHNIQUE: The surgical area is aseptically prepared. Margins at least 2 cm beyond the limit of the mass are identified and outlined using the CO_2 laser in pulse mode (Figure CS20-1). Directing the handpiece perpendicular to the skin, laser energy is applied at the correct focal distance for vaporization to make an incision. Once good edges are produced, the surgeon should retract the mass and undermine it, directing the handpiece parallel to the dermis. After saving the specimen for histopathology, the laser is prepared to use the scanner. The scanner is directed perpendicular to the surgical area and all tissue with atypical appearance is ablated. Care should be taken to attempt to leave the nerve and vessels in this region (Figure CS20-2). After each pass any char should be wiped away and the area re-evaluated for residual atypical tissue.

COMMENTS: This technique can be used when the client refuses more radical excision due to unfavorable post-operative cosmetic appearance.

CLOSURE: Standard two-layer simple interrupted pattern closure using 2-0 absorbable monofilament material to appose the subcutis and 2-0 non-absorbable monofilament for skin closure (Figure CS20-3).

POST-OP EVALUATION: Histopathology is best indicator of tumor-free margins. Evaluate buffy coat for circulating mast cells. Consider ultrasonogram study of liver and spleen. Internist may recommend bone marrow biopsy. Consultation with a veterinary oncologist is indicated.

FOLLOW-UP: The patient is evaluated fourteen days later and sutures are removed at this time. Six-month re-checks are recommended.

Case Study 21
Canine Cystotomy

4-year-old male neutered Lhasa-Apso, presented for multiple urinary calculi.

PROCEDURE: CO_2 laser-assisted cystotomy.

ANESTHESIA: Pre-medicated with medetomedine, butorphanol, and glycopyrrolate. Mask induction with isoflurane in oxygen. Maintenance of general anesthesia via endotracheal tube.

EQUIPMENT: 12-Watt or 20-Watt CO_2 Novapulse™ laser, suction, and irrigation.

LASER SETTINGS:
   Spot Diameter: 0.8 mm
   Power Output: 10 to 12 W
   Beam Output: CW

TECHNIQUE: Once the abdomen is opened, the urinary bladder is identified and isolated with sterile moistened laparotomy sponges. A stay suture is placed to anchor the bladder in one fixed area. Creating a cystotomy incision also will cause the urinary bladder to contract and become smaller after the urine is emptied (Figure CS21-1). A sterile assistant is prepared with suction to remove any urine immediately before it contaminates the surgical field. Smoke evacuation accompanies the laser incision as well. The bladder is incised in a relatively avascular area near the apex on the ventral side, if possible. The CO_2 laser is used to vaporize a hole in the bladder serosa and mucosa. The air forced through a hollow, flexible waveguide will slightly fill the bladder when the mucosa has been ablated. At this exact moment the surgeon and assistant work together to extend the incision and avoid urine contamination as the bladder empties. The full thickness incision is continued to a length that will accommodate the entry of a suction tip (Figure CS21-2). The bladder is emptied of urine and the procedure continues as indicated. A sterile rigid endoscope may be introduced within the cystotomy incision to aid in the detection and removal of all cystic calculi.

COMMENTS: Using a CO_2 laser for this procedure greatly reduces post-operative discomfort and minimizes post-operative hematuria.

CLOSURE: Standard double-row inverting pattern using absorbable monofilament suture material (Figure CS21-3).

POST-OP EVALUATION: Assess normal bladder function, renal function, sepsis, hydration, and patient comfort.

FOLLOW-UP: Two weeks later, following a course of antibiotic therapy and appropriate dietary modification.

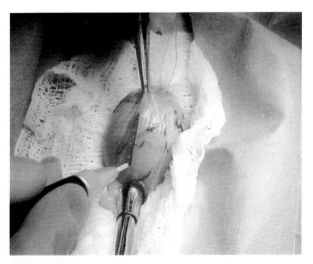

Figure CS21-1

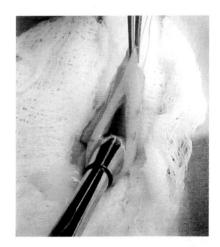

Figure CS21-2

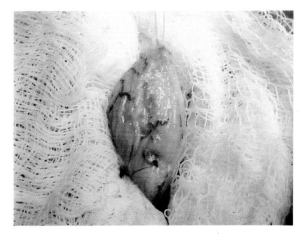

Figure CS21-3

Case Study 22
Feline Myringotomy

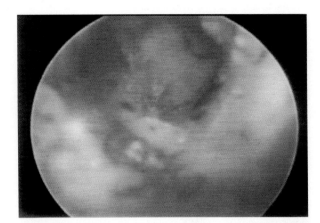

Figure CS22-1

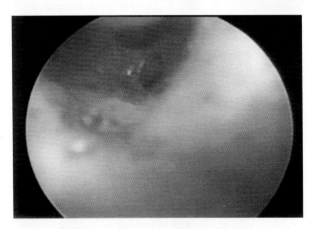

Figure CS22-2

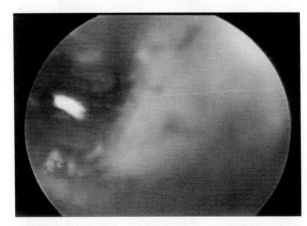

Figure CS22-3

5-year-old male neutered Himalayan cat, presented for a history of chronic otitis.

PROCEDURE: Otoendoscopic CO_2 laser-assisted myringotomy.

ANESTHESIA: Pre-medicated with medetomedine, butorphanol, and glycopyrrolate. Mask induction with isoflurane in oxygen. Maintenance of general anesthesia via endotracheal tube.

EQUIPMENT: 12-Watt or 20-Watt CO_2 Novapulse™ laser, video otoendoscope, flexible laser tip, 3.5 Fr tomcat catheter, suction and flushing device.

LASER SETTINGS:
 Spot Diameter: 0.8 mm
 Power Output: 4 to 6 W
 Beam Output: 100 msec to 500 msec CW

TECHNIQUE: A clean ear is first achieved (Figure CS22-1). The flexible laser tip is advanced through the working channel of a video otoendoscope. A single burst of energy is targeted at the tympanum to create a window through which internal pressures are relieved. It is directed at the 5 o'clock position in the left ear, and at the 7 o'clock position in the right ear. In some cases, multiple bursts may be needed to perforate the tympanum in a precise and controlled fashion (Figure CS22-2).

COMMENTS: Immediately following myringotomy, it is not unusual for pus to emerge from the bulla. This may be sampled for bacterial culture and sensitivity (Figure CS22-3). The bulla is repeatedly flushed with warm sterile saline passed through a 3.5 Fr tomcat catheter. When the middle ear is clean and dry, a small volume of a fluroquinolone antibiotic and steroidal anti-inflammatory mixture is infused within the bulla using a new 3.5 Fr tomcat catheter (we use three-fourths cc Baytril™ and one-fourth cc Synotic™).

This procedure may also be performed very nicely with a 980 nm diode laser using a 600μm diameter fiber to deliver laser energy in contact mode to the pars tensa of the tympanum. We generally use three to eight pulses of 5 W to 8 W(for 0.1 s at a duty factor of 50%) in a fluid medium. In cases where stenosis or swelling prevents the use of a CO_2 laser, the diode laser is a superior alternative. The pressure of the fluid within the horizontal ear canal both dilates the canal and provides for greater magnification through the video-otoendoscope.

CLOSURE: None. Avoid any more fluid in ear canal for five more days.

POST-OP EVALUATION: Observe for vestibular signs, recurrent otitis, or pain. These pre-operative symptoms are generally relieved by the myringotomy procedure.

FOLLOW-UP: In one week, only the infusion procedure should be repeated; however, the myringotomy should not need to be re-done. Longer period of time for follow-up may require a myringotomy to be re-performed if the fenestration has healed and sealed.

Case Study 23
Canine Skin Incision

7-year-old female spayed Collie, presented for surgical removal of a lipoma.

PROCEDURE: Skin incision.

ANESTHESIA: Pre-medicated with medetomedine, butorphanol, and glycopyrrolate. Mask induction with isoflurane in oxygen. Maintenance of general anesthesia via endotracheal tube.

EQUIPMENT: 20-Watt CO_2 Novapulse™ laser with straight handpiece and 0.4 mm metal or gold tip.

LASER SETTINGS
    Spot Diameter: 0.4 mm
    Power Output: 6 to 8 W
    Beam Output: Pulsed pattern C-3, SP

TECHNIQUE: Tension is applied across the planned incision site using digital manipulation (Figure CS23-1). The focused tip is held so that the laser energy is delivered at the focal distance from the target. The handpiece is held perpendicular to the target, and the incision is made with hand speed appropriate for tissue separation under tension. Using a pulsed pattern allows the tissue to cool between laser energy bursts, thus minimizing char. Once completed, the edges are wiped free of excessive char using sterile, saline-soaked gauze (Figure CS23-2).

COMMENTS: The incision is clean, dry, and not painful to the patient upon anesthetic recovery. The superpulse temporal pattern is an ideal setting for skin incisions. If available, the superpulse setting also can be pulsed for a greater reduction in char formation (Figure CS23-3).

CLOSURE: Adequate subcuticular sutures are required. Outer layer closure may be accomplished with simple interrupted non-absorbable suture, or with a surgical tissue adhesive.

POST-OP EVALUATION: The patient should not be interested in grooming the area. The suture line requires fourteen days to heal.

FOLLOW-UP: If sutures are required to be removed after fourteen days, the tensile strength of the healed incision should be evaluated prior to removal.

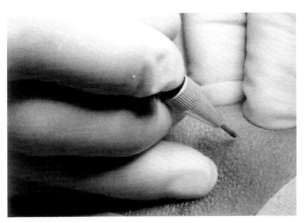

Figure CS23-1

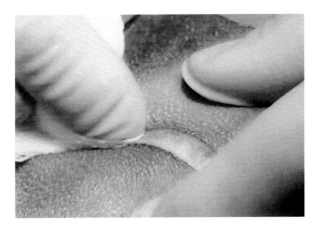

Figure CS23-2

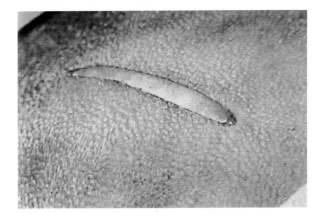

Figure CS23-3

Case Study 24
Canine Ovariohysterectomy

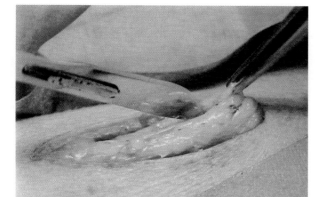

Figure CS24-1

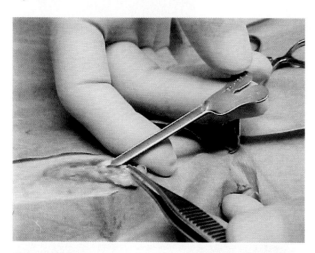

Figure CS24-2

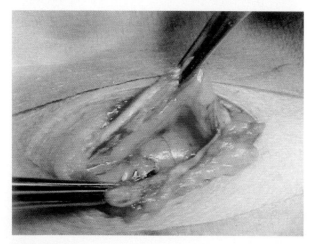

Figure CS24-3

6-month-old female Golden Retriever, presented for spay.

PROCEDURE: Abdominal approach for canine ovariohysterectomy.

ANESTHESIA: Pre-medicated with medetomedine, butorphanol, and glycopyrrolate. Mask induction with isoflurane in oxygen. Maintenance of general anesthesia via endotracheal tube.

EQUIPMENT: 12-Watt or 20-Watt CO_2 Novapulse™ laser, non-reflective backstop.

LASER SETTINGS:
  Spot Diameter: 0.4 mm
  Power Output: 6 to 8 W
  Beam Output: Pulsed pattern for skin incision, CW to continue the abdominal incision

TECHNIQUE: A skin incision is made and the subcutaneous tissues are cleanly dissected from the linea alba. The abdominal muscles and peritoneum are tented up with forceps and a single cranial stab incision is created with a scalpel blade (Figure CS24-1). A linear non-reflective metallic object (grooved director) is introduced into the abdominal incision to serve as a backstop for the CO_2 laser-assisted continuation of the incision. All internal structures must be protected from stray laser beams. Inadvertent lasing of the spleen, bladder, or mesenteric blood vessels could prove disastrous and should be avoided. The abdomen is incised using 0.4 mm tip, 6 W to 8 W CW over the backstop, which is lifted upward to tense the targeted muscles that are vaporized (Figure CS24-2). Any char is wiped away from the clean and dry muscle edges (Figure CS24-3). The procedure is then continued as previously performed by the surgeon's routine technique.

COMMENTS: The use of a CO_2 laser for the skin incision and abdominal incision greatly reduces the pain and discomfort associated with recovery from major abdominal surgery.

CLOSURE: Three-layer closure. Surgical adhesive may be used if desired to minimize use of external sutures.

POST-OP EVALUATION: Incision should be clean, dry, and intact. Subcuticular sutures and tissue adhesive may be used instead of outer-layer sutures.

FOLLOW-UP: Recheck and suture removal in seven to ten days.

Case Study 25
Feline Thyroidectomy

11-year-old female spayed hyperthyroid Domestic Shorthair, presented for bilateral thyroid lobe excision.

PROCEDURE: Laser-assisted hemostasis of supporting blood vessels during bilateral thyroidectomy.

ANESTHESIA: Pre-medicated with medetomedine, butorphanol, and glycopyrrolate. Mask induction with isoflurane in oxygen. Maintenance of general anesthesia via endotracheal tube.

EQUIPMENT: 12-Watt or 20-Watt CO_2 Novapulse™ laser, sterile cotton–tipped applicators.

LASER SETTINGS:
  Spot Diameter: 0.3 mm
  Power Output: 2 to 5 W
  Beam Output: Pulsed pattern for skin incision, CW for vessel
    vaporization

TECHNIQUE: A ventral incision is made through the skin overlying the caudal larynx. The sternohyoideus and sternothyroideus muscles are longitudinally separated and the trachea is exposed (Figure CS25-1). The caudal thyroid vein is located and isolated using forceps and a moistened, sterile, cotton-tipped applicator. Once the underlying structures are identified and protected, the vessel is transected and sealed with the laser using a defocused beam (Figure CS25-2). Sterile, moistened, cotton-tipped applicators are used to very gently tease the thyroid gland free from its connective tissue attachments. Care must also be taken to avoid excessive disturbance of the cranial thyroid artery, especially when bilateral thyroidectomy is required. Vaporizing the cranial thyroid artery completes the thyroid lobectomy. Gentle traction facilitates separation of the thyroid from the parathyroid gland (Figure CS25-3).

COMMENTS: When bilateral thyroidectomy is performed, it is advisable to stage the procedures thirty days apart, or use dihydrotachysterol to minimize the potential for hypoparathyroidism. An autogenous parathyroid graft may be planted within the sternohyoid muscle to preserve normal calcium metabolism.

CLOSURE: The muscle layers are closed with 4-0 monofilament absorbable suture material, and the skin is closed with surgical adhesive.

POST-OP EVALUATION: Assess serum calcium levels forty-eight hours following recovery.

FOLLOW-UP: Patient should be euthyroid within two to four weeks.

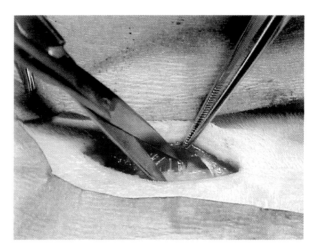

Figure CS25-1

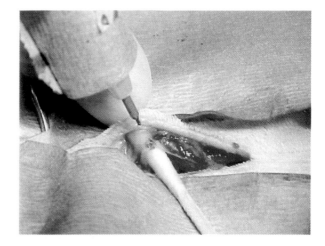

Figure CS25-2

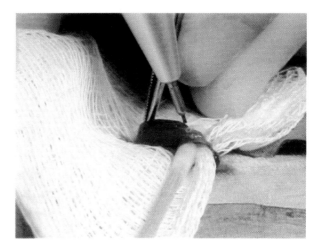

Figure CS25-3

Case Study 26
Feline Tail Amputation

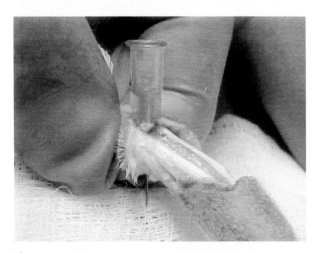

Figure CS26-1

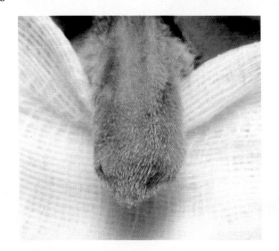

Figure CS26-2

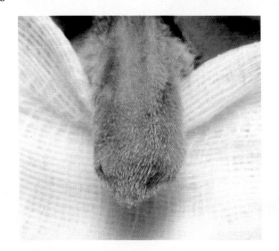

Figure CS26-3

4-year-old male neutered Domestic Shorthair, presented for necrotizing and gangrenous tail injury.

PROCEDURE: Disarticulation of caudal vertebrae proximal to injury site using CO_2 laser.

ANESTHESIA: Pre-medicated with medetomedine, butorphanol, and glycopyrrolate. Mask induction with isoflurane in oxygen. Maintenance of general anesthesia via endotracheal tube.

EQUIPMENT: 20-Watt CO_2 Novapulse™ laser with straight handpiece.

LASER SETTINGS:
   Spot Diameter: 0.4 mm for skin incision, 0.8 mm for disarticulation
   Power Output: 6 to 8 W skin incision, 8 to 12 W disarticulation
   Beam Output: Pulsed pattern skin incision, CW disarticulation

TECHNIQUE: A dorsal and a ventral skin incision is made using a 0.4 mm tip, 6 W to 8W CW SP. The incisions are made in the shape of a "V" so that the posterior edge of the incision is pointed, and the proximal edges of the incision meet at the level of the intended separation of caudal vertebrae (Figure CS26-1). Any char is aggressively wiped away with moistened sterile gauze. The surgeon should identify the intervertebral space using a sterile 25 gauge needle to demonstrate the joint (Figure CS26-2). Under tension, vaporize connective tissue, ligaments, artery vein, and nerve at the level of the joint using 0.8 mm tip, 8 W to 12 W CW in short bursts of 100 to 500 msec duration. Avoid charring the distal edge of the remaining caudal vertebra. The incision is lavaged with sterile saline prior to closure.

COMMENTS: When required because of trauma, unresolved deformation, or tumors and their consequential diphtheritic suppuration, amputation of the tail is a humane procedure that relieves pain and eliminates sepsis. Antibiotics are dispensed for ten days following the procedure.

CLOSURE: Simple interrupted steel or monofilament suture material. Closure should approximate a conical shape (Figure CS26-3). An Elizabethan collar should be worn to prevent self-mutilation and/or early suture removal by the patient.

POST-OP EVALUATION: Incision should be clean and dry and not swollen. When the patient sits, the tail should not drive directly downward.

FOLLOW-UP: Suture removal in ten to fourteen days.

Case Study 27
Canine Cherry-Eye Repair

6-month-old male Lhasa Apso, presented for neuter and correction of inflamed nictitans gland.

PROCEDURE: CO_2 laser hemostasis of supporting blood vessel as a modification of Morgan's pocket technique.

ANESTHESIA: Pre-medicated with medetomedine, butorphanol, and glycopyrrolate. Mask induction with isoflurane in oxygen. Maintenance of general anesthesia via endotracheal tube.

EQUIPMENT: 20-Watt CO_2 Novapulse™ laser with straight handpiece, iris scissors.

LASER SETTINGS:
  Spot Diameter: 0.3 mm
  Power Output: 2 to 4 W
  Beam Output: CW

TECHNIQUE: There is an appreciable engorged conjunctival vessel that supports the gland of the nictitans (Figure CS27-1). There is generally a great deal of hemorrhage that obscures the field when it is transected to create the pocket that receives the tucked-in nictitans gland. Prior to using the laser, ensure the exposed structures of the globe are protected from stray laser beams. Vaporize this vessel with CO_2 laser energy through a 0.3mm tip using 2 W to 4 W CW (Figure CS27-2). The incision is then continued around the inflamed gland (with the SP setting, if available) to minimize char. After wiping away any char, the bulbar conjunctival pocket is developed by blunt dissection using iris scissors.

COMMENTS: Morgan, et al. (1993) described this "pocket technique" for correction of inflamed gland of nictitans as 95% successful in all breeds. This is our preferred technique as simplified with a CO_2 laser. The key advantage to using a laser in this technique is hemostasis (Figure CS27-3).

CLOSURE: Monofilament 4-0 or 5-0 absorbable material. Knots should be tied on palpebral surface of third eyelid. Two lines of continuous inverting suture hold the inflamed gland within a pocket created within the bulbar conjunctiva. Ophthalmic antibiotic ointment is applied twice daily for five days following recovery.

POST-OP EVALUATION: Sutures should not irritate cornea, and patient should be comfortable and have pleasant appearance one week later at final recheck.

FOLLOW-UP: None

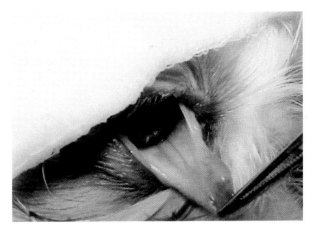

Figure CS27-1

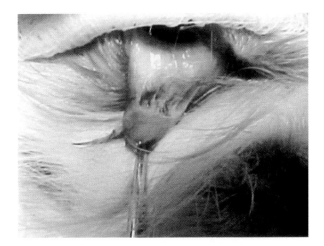

Figure CS27-2

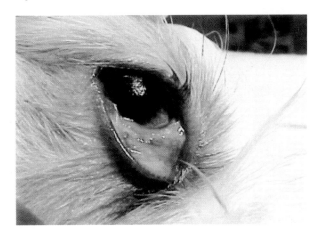

Figure CS27-3

Case Study 28
Canine Stenotic Nares Repair

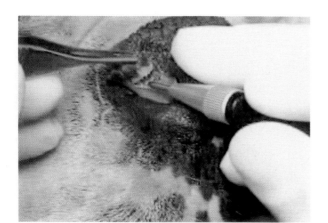

Figure CS28-1

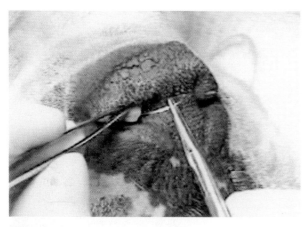

Figure CS28-2

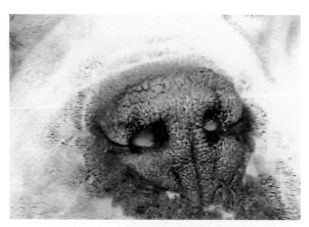

Figure CS28-3

6-year-old male neutered Bulldog, presented for breathing problems associated with brachycephalic breed upper airway syndrome, requiring correction of elongated soft palate, tonsillectomy, and opening stenotic nares.

PROCEDURE: Vertical nare resection using CO_2 laser as the incising instrument.

ANESTHESIA: Pre-medicated with medetomedine, butorphanol, and glycopyrrolate. Mask induction with isoflurane in oxygen. Maintenance of general anesthesia via endotracheal tube.

EQUIPMENT: 20-Watt CO_2 Novapulse™ laser with straight handpiece, protective patient eye shields.

LASER SETTINGS:
  Spot Diameter: 0.3 mm in small patients, 0.4 mm in larger patients
  Power Output: 2 to 4 W with a 0.3 mm tip, 5 to 7 W with a 0.4 mm tip
  Beam Output: Pulsed pattern for initial marking, CW for nare resection

TECHNIQUE: The surgeon envisions the final nasal opening as a circular conduit for airflow. To do this, a conical, wedge-shaped portion of the stenotic nare is removed using a 0.3 mm tip, 2 W to 4 W or 0.4 mm tip, 5 W to 7 W. Pulsing the laser allows the surgeon to precisely indicate the desired amount of tissue planned for excision. Continue the incision of the nostril from the philtrum toward the alar fold to make the circular shape complete. To excise the redundant tissue that causes the stenosis, apply tension as the laser dissects deep into the nostril space using CW setting (Figure CS28-1). Any remaining tissue in this area may also be excised until the surgeon is satisfied sufficient tissue has been removed to ameliorate the stenosis. There should be no bleeding in this highly vascular area; however, if minor hemorrhage occurs, the surgeon should apply a defocused low-power laser beam for hemostasis.

COMMENTS: Owners should be instructed to keep the area clean and moist for several days to prevent buildup of mucus or scabs.

CLOSURE: The nasal mucosa is sutured to the keratinized epithelium using 3-0 or 4-0 monofilament absorbable suture material (Figure CS28-2).

POST-OP EVALUATION: The new nares should be symmetrical and open and have a pleasing appearance (Figure CS28-3).

FOLLOW-UP: If there is a need to remove the sutures, it should be postponed until complete healing occurs, after 21-day post-op.

Case Study 29
Feline Hypergingival Odontoclastic Lesion

7-year-old female Domestic Shorthair, presented for hyperplastic gingival flap overlying grade-one odontoclastic lesion repair (Figure CS29-1).

PROCEDURE: Excision of hyperplastic gingival tissue. Exposure of odontoclastic lesion and glass ionomer filling.

ANESTHESIA: Pre-medicated with medetomedine, butorphanol, and glycopyrrolate. Mask induction with isoflurane in oxygen. Maintenance of general anesthesia via endotracheal tube.

EQUIPMENT: 20-Watt CO_2 Novapulse™ laser with straight handpiece and 0.4 mm metal or gold tip.

LASER SETTINGS:
  Spot Diameter: 0.4 mm
  Power Output: 6 W
  Beam Output: CW

TECHNIQUE: The affected tooth and gingival tissue are cleaned of any calculi or debris. The hyperplastic gingival tissue is elevated away from the tooth. A periosteal elevator is used to elevate the gingival tissue and act as a backstop to protect the underlying tooth anatomy. The laser tip is directed perpendicular to the hyperplastic gingival tissue and the tissue excised at the level of the adjoining gingival surface (Figure CS29-2). If bleeding is noted, the laser tip is defocused and a single pulse of energy is directed near the vessel. Any char is gently wiped away and the odontoclastic lesion is evaluated and prepared for filling with a glass ionomer-curing compound (Figure CS29-3). The tooth is then polished.

COMMENTS: The great advantage of CO_2 laser energy use in the oral cavity is the reduction in bleeding and increased ability to provide a clean and dry environment in which to work. Care must be taken to protect the endotracheal tube from direct exposure to laser energy.

CLOSURE: None is typically required. If any gingival tissue needs to be closed, 3-0 or 4-0 chromic gut is recommended.

POST-OP EVALUATION: Recheck tooth and gingival tissue post-recovery.

FOLLOW-UP: Recheck tooth and gingival tissue in fourteen days.

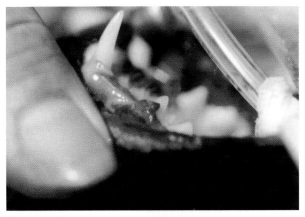

Figure CS29-1

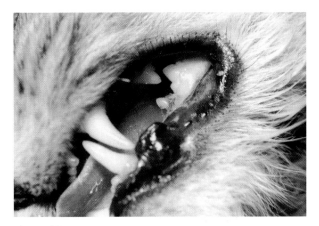

Figure CS29-2

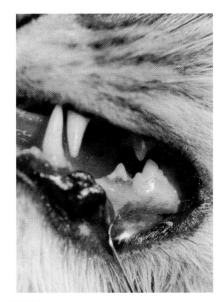

Figure CS29-3

Case Study 30
Feline Faucitis Stomatitis Treatment

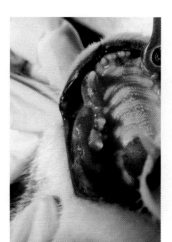

Figure CS30-1

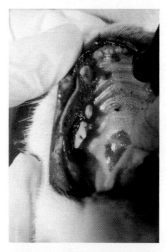

Figure CS30-2

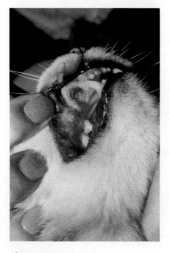

Figure CS30-3

5-year-old male Domestic Shorthair, presented for ablation of severe purulent faucitis-stomatitis (Figure CS30-1).

PROCEDURE: Ablation of inflamed gingival tissue using pattern scanner.

ANESTHESIA: Pre-medicated with medetomedine, butorphanol, and glycopyrrolate. Mask induction with isoflurane in oxygen. Maintenance of general anesthesia via endotracheal tube.

EQUIPMENT: 20-Watt CO_2 Novapulse™ laser, mechanical scanner with 3 mm pattern scans.

LASER SETTINGS:
  Spot Diameter: 3 mm pattern scan using a 0.8 mm daisywheel spot
  Power Output: 10 W
  Beam Output: SP or CW

TECHNIQUE: The oral cavity is flushed and the affected area cleaned with an antiseptic gel or cleaning solution. The endotracheal tube is protected from exposure to laser energy. The scanning tip is directed perpendicular to the affected tissue and laser energy delivered to ablate abnormal gingival tissue. In areas where the tooth is present a periosteal elevator protects the underlying tooth enamel. It is important to wipe away any char formed after each pass with the scanner (Figure CS30-2). Wiping with a 0.9% NaCl-soaked gauze also serves the additional purpose of identifying any remaining friable bleeding gingival tissue. The area affected is re-treated until there is no bleeding back from the gingival surface. At this point any remaining char is wiped away and the area liberally flushed with sterile 0.9% NaCl.

COMMENTS: Faucitis-stomatitis can be manifested from immune-related disorders (hyper-responsive) or primary bacterial infection (hypo-responsive). Treatment of the former with laser energy provides palliative relief from pain and swelling. Recurrence at the surgical site is likely. Treatment of the latter is usually curative provided a proper culture and sensitivity has been done and appropriate antibiotic therapy instituted. We like a fluroquinolone and metronidazole (15 mg/kg/day) combination therapy.

CLOSURE: None. Topical coating of 2% lidocaine is recommended upon completion of the procedure.

POST-OP EVALUATION: Normal gingival tissue and or some fibrocartilagenous scar tissue should be noted in place of the inflamed gingival tissue within seven to ten days of treatment (Figure CS30-3). Significant reduction in pain and odor should be noted almost immediately upon recovery.

FOLLOW-UP: These cases should be closely monitored for recurrence.

Index